The Body Within

The Body Within

Within

Who are We Really?

Marie Knoetig

Disclaimer

A new method is introduced. It is called the Body Within. This is continuing research. I am not a medical doctor and I do not practice medicine. Healing is based on the energy field that connects us to the universe.

I do not diagnose or prescribe medication. I assist people in correcting energy imbalances in the different fields of their being to release negative energy. When the energy of the body is balanced, the body's natural energy heals itself.

All healing promoted in this book and my work is self-healing. I strongly recommend that clients continue to see their regular medical practitioners and use my work as a complement to their healing.

The methods and theories in this book have worked for me and my healing. They may or may not be right for you and your healing. You need to use your own judgment in exploring and using any exercises or techniques in this book.

If you are concerned about any health issue you may have, please see a qualified physician for guidance.

Edited by Christine Corriveau
Cover by Cyndi Carr
Picture by Bob Clegg

This book is dedicated to my brother, Steve.

Life has handed us many challenges. The one constant in my life has been that you have always had my back and I have always had yours. The security you have afforded me through the years is the main reason I have become the strong woman I am today! I am forever grateful to have you in my life.

Love you!

Table of Contents

Introduction

It's difficult for me to explain something that comes so natural to me. When someone is on my treatment table, I am able to tap into the life force energy of their body. As I do this, I am able to see or sense their energy anatomy and any blockages in their energy that might be inhibiting the person's healing. It could be physical or emotional imbalances in their life, and on a more specific level, imbalances in the muscular skeletal system and any dysfunctions that are keeping the body from healing.

What do I mean by this? When I look at an individual I not only see them lying in front of me on the table. I see an energy imprint on their physical body along with other layers of energy. It's like someone puts a clear piece of plastic in front of their physical body and marks lines and spots on it to show where the dysfunction in the tissue lies. Here's an example. If you come in and see me because you have had right shoulder pain for two years and you don't remember ever having a specific injury to the shoulder, and physical therapy and any advice the doctors have given you has not resolved the issue, I am able to see or sense these imprints energetically and, a lot of times, figure out what is causing the shoulder pain. Sometimes, I might sense it is caused by the opposite knee and a dysfunction in your gait (your manner of walking or running). It may be you had your appendix removed and I see or sense some of the scar tissue is now restricting you from fully lifting your arm from your midsection of your torso, which causes pressure on your shoulder joint, or you might have had a torn ACL (ligament) repair in the opposite knee six or more years prior to the shoulder pain onset.

You see, every time we sustain an injury to our body, the body immediately puts up a wall of protection to protect the injury. This wall not only shuts down body movement in the area of the injury, but it also limits movement in other areas of the body that affect the injury.   In time, as you heal the injury, you regain a good portion of movement back, but a lot of times we still have some dysfunction in the area of the injury or any areas of movement in the body that pull on the injury while healing. This is what I see energetically, the left over debris, as I call it. If we don't clean up and regain full function from a previous injury, it starts to create blockages in our energy imprint, as well as the fluid gait of our body. This can cause new injuries to not heal quickly or properly, or even aid in creating an injury due to what is called "cumulative trauma disorder"[1]. The fascinating part is, everyone has lived their lives in a completely different manner so one person's body does not have the same injuries as another person. Sometimes, in order to help a new injury heal, there is a pattern in an old injury or dysfunction that needs to be found. By using the energy as a tool, I am able to see or sense your energy imprint of

---

[1] Cumulative trauma disorder identifies a large group of conditions that result from traumatizing the body in either a minute or major way over a period of time.

past injuries to help you resolve the shoulder issue after we figure out what is slowing the healing of the shoulder.

From there, I am self-taught in hands on energy release of tissue restrictions, using my intuition and my knowledge of how the body moves from my training with exercise and my degree in Exercise Science, I am able to help facilitate the body in energetically releasing these restrictions and help the individual regain mobility back to the limited joints. From there, I refer the client to a massage therapist, chiropractor, osteopath, or even to see their primary care physician to refer them to physical therapy if needed. This is only one of the many intuitive functions I am able to help clients with. Each session is individualized, so when the client comes in I am able to connect to their own personal energy field what I call the Body Within. I believe the Body Within is the true essence of who we are. As soon as I connect to it energetically their Body Within guides me through the endless possibilities in their healing. Sometimes during the session we key in on the energetic blockages in the physical body, sometimes it's emotional, and sometimes we work with the energies that are creating an imbalance in the client's life. These could be stress, anger, sometimes negativity, or even grief. It could be grief they have not healed from or if someone close to them has died and neither one (client or deceased) have healed. This can cause an imbalance in each person's energies. There are so many ways the body struggles to heal, and working with these reasons and helping the client create balance aids the individual in healing.

3

Now that I explained all that, you might be thinking, "Does she consider herself a psychic or medium, or someone like that?" I would answer that with a definite "NO"! What I consider myself is a person that is sensitive to the subtle energies that we all are made of. Someone who has, through their own healing, tapped in to a small piece of the endless possibilities we all are as humans. By being balanced in life and present with each client along with the many skills I have acquired in my life, I am able to see what most of us miss happening around us on a daily basis. Being open and balanced has helped me become a facilitator for those who want to learn more about their own body and the life force energy that is us. In doing this, I am able to help the individual create healing for themselves.

This self-taught technique also aids in many other health issues such as autoimmune, arthritis, cancer, etc. Helping the individual with energy balancing and teaching them about their energy anatomy aids them in their everyday living. It also helps them in making choices and becoming more aware of the imbalances in energy around them, whether it's work, family, diet, rest, friends, or even outside energetic influences.

My goal in writing this book is to show you how I interpret the energy anatomy of the body and how to use it to self-heal your body, mind, and spirit. How the choices we make every day, like what to eat, how much rest do I need, do I work too much, to making medical choices in an overwhelming system of Western medicine[2] and alternative medicine[3], not only serve us now, but they serve us when our journey is over and we are ready to die.

Last year, 55 billion dollars was spent by Medicare on doctors and hospital bills during the last two months of a patient's life. (CBSnews.com, 2009) The unfortunate part is that most of that money was not targeted to aid in creating a more peaceful death. It was used for treating symptoms or prolonging life. Unfortunately, when it comes time to end our journey, something we will all experience, most of us have no idea how to listen to our bodies and allow the natural process of death to occur. Instead of allowing one of the most natural things to happen to us, we fear it and make choices to stay until we have our last breath, no matter the quality of life.

We are taught many things in our life, from the time of birth on how to live, get a good job, plan for our future, etc. The one thing, as a society, we really don't talk about much, or even teach about, is how to die. Ironically, it is the one guarantee in life we will all experience. What would we teach, if we were to start to introduce the topic of death in schools? Do we even have a healthy way of perceiving death in society?

---

[2] A system in which medical doctors and other healthcare professions (such as nurses, pharmacists, and therapists) treat symptoms and disease using drugs, or surgery, rehabilitation, etc. Considered mainstream medicine.

[3] A variety of therapeutic or preventative healthcare practices such as homeopathy, naturopathy, chiropractic, and herbal medicines that do not follow generally accepted medical methods.

The Conversation Project is trying to open that line of thinking. The project began in 2010, when Ellen Goodman and a group of people gathered to share stories of good deaths and bad deaths (as they refer to them) within their own circle of loved ones. As they compiled stories, the one common theme in the good deaths was when loved ones held many conversations with the dying individual. This seemed to lessen the fear and help the loved one choose their end of life wishes. They found that these deaths tended to be more peaceful. It's an amazing project that is getting people to talk about death. If you would like more information about the Conversation Project please visit their website at www.theconversationprogect.org

My goal is to take this conversation one step further and show you that if you can learn to get in touch with what I call your Body Within, now, while you are living, then you too can have a peaceful perception of death and dying and maybe even choose the timing.

What do I interpret as the Body Within? The true essence of who we are. It's that good angel/bad angel on your shoulder we see in cartoons except it's the true essence of who we are. Our Body Within - good angel - argues with, what I call, our created reality (or misinterpreted reality) - bad angel. Our created reality is what we *believe* to be true, or what we *think* we want, or the *beliefs* that have been imposed upon us by society, family, or others in our lives.

The Body Within is our good cop, and our mediator, to police ourselves – to help us see what's really happening around us, not what we interpret as happening - and help us be the best we can be. It helps us know how to eat and sleep right, exercise, to reduce stress, and learn what makes us happy with family, careers, hobbies, friends, etc. The good angel is always alerting us if we need help in these areas. It's up to us to learn to listen.

The key to listening is to learn to balance ourselves and our lives around us so we can start to hear all the amazing messages, intuitively, just waiting for us. What do I consider balance and why is it so important? Balance is the power of three – body, mind, and spirit. I believe we should balance all three. I believe they are all equal! Yes, I did say equal! So, if all three are equal, that means you should pay equal attention to your body, mind, and your spirit every day! Yes, every day! What that means is every day you should check in with all three. Maybe, thirty minutes a night before bed. See how your body is doing. Does it need anything? Are you feeling tired? Maybe, some stretching? Was your nutrition sound today? Did you get any exercise today? Do you need exercise? Can you do better tomorrow? Then you should think about your day. Check in to see if it was busy, manageable, etc. How did you handle issues that came your way? Did you see them clearly? Were you tired and unfocused? If you were how was your nutrition? Were you sharp and on task? Next, your Body Within (your spirit), did you hear it at all? Was it alerting you to anything? Did you listen or did you overrule it? My challenge to you, as I give you the tools, is this: Try balancing all three and see if it has a positive effect on you and your daily living.

When you work to balance yourself it creates quiet in your energy, this will help you to hear the Body Within. As you listen to the Body Within, life becomes less complicated and the knowing inside teaches you how to live a truly fulfilling and productive life.

The most important part of connecting with your Body Within is it not only teaches us how to live, it teaches us that we're all here for a limited amount of time. This journey will end. The choices we make about how to live not only serve us now, but they serve us when we're ready to die. Think about the Conservation Project. If just a conversation has the potential to change a bad death to a good death, then connecting to your Body Within can give you the power to have the conversation with yourself. That puts you in the driver's seat. I know this sounds crazy – that we actually might have control over how we die, but I believe if you learn to listen now, you will automatically listen then!

Start reading and I'll do my best to share with you what I know. I'll show you that, if you balance your life and get to know your Body Within, the true essence of who you are, you can and will change your life for the here and now -- and the hereafter.

Happy reading!
Marie ☺

My Story

I grew up in New England, in a family with nine siblings and a strong French-Canadian and Catholic background. I made many wrong decisions growing up and learned some pretty hard lessons.

About 30 years into my journey, my life ended up in a very challenging place. I had a husband, three children, a job, and house to tend to after having many knee surgeries, c-sections, a severe injury to my shoulder girdle and all the muscles supporting it. The right side of my body was very weak due to the nerve damage of the shoulder and all the scar tissue in my upper body. This affected my gait and any physical activity of any kind. I also suffered from severe asthma, allergies, and environmental sensitivities. The many doctors and specialist I had seen said they were doing all they could to manage my heath issues but they did not have any answers to help me regain total health. I was 30 years old and I found myself in a position many other people find themselves in, having chronic health issues that have been treated and managed but deemed unfixable in the scope of Western medicine.

I felt I had two choices. I could either try to live in chronic pain and with chronic illness, or find a way to help myself heal. Having exhausted all the resources I knew of at the time, I had one love in my life besides my husband and children, and that was exercise. If I was unable to find answers in Western medicine, then exercise was going to fix me or, at least, keep me sane.

I enrolled in college in an Exercise Science program. I felt like the more I learned about my body and how it should work, the better chance I had of getting it to work. I was the most alert and attentive student in the program, and I was blessed with a professor who felt that no question was a dumb one. As I learned kinesiology, the study of human movement, I learned it from the inside of the book to the inside of my body. If a muscle pulled on another muscle, I focused until I could feel how the pull felt in my own body. This resulted in two realizations. First, I became very sensitive to how the body moved and how the physical structure is so specific and amazing. Second, I became aware of how critical my situation was and how challenging it was going to be to reach my goal of self-healing.

It was then that I met a physical therapist trained in integrative manual therapy. I was referred to her by a physiatrist – a doctor of physical therapy. The doctor said I had so much belly scarring (from three consecutive C-sections in five years), and lack of upper body function (a paralyzed shoulder due to complications following shoulder surgery), that this physical therapist offered the only modality he knew that might give me some relief. The doctor called it integrative manual therapy. The doctor explained to me that integrative manual therapy is a gentle, hands-on approach to restoring posture and allowing optimal movement to return. This helps in restoring health and wellness for the whole body. It

10

addresses the relationship between the bones, joints, ligaments, muscles, fascia, arteries, veins, lymphatic system, brain, and organs. It was a fresh look at a complicated problem.

I had never heard of integrative therapy, and knew nothing about it. All I knew was it felt right, so I decided to check it out. Little did I know it would change my life!

As we started to work together, the physical therapist showed me some techniques I could try on myself. She said I had so much scarring and muscle dysfunction I could work on myself for a very long time and only break the surface. The more I learned to do this therapy myself, the better chance I had to reverse the damage. As she showed me how to release tissue restrictions, I would come back and show her how I figured out a different way to do the techniques she showed me. I was not really aware that I should not know a different way. My agenda was to get better, so I hadn't really thought about what was happening!

The more techniques she showed me, the more I figured out a different way of using them for myself. I would just sit quietly and focus on what she showed me, and I would see in my mind a whole new way to approach it. She never commented on how I was helping myself, she would just smile. As my therapy came to a close, due to insurance limitations, her parting words were, "Keep reading about energy medicine and practicing. You will be teaching me in a few years." I thought she was absolutely crazy. But, in retrospect, I think she knew I had begun to sense the energy and was able to work with it.

From the time I left Linda's care, I began my journey in hands-on energy release of tissue restrictions. Using my own intuition and my knowledge of how the body moves from my training with exercise and my exercise science, I was developing my own method to help myself and, eventually, others.

About three years later, we met up at a conference and ended up working out of the same office for a while – and we were and still are co-treating patients to help them get the best outcome. It was amazing to brainstorm with her on a regular basis. She was an integral part of my journey. She was able to see more in me than most and helped me to see it myself. So Linda, thank you. You're awesome!

As time went on, I was working in a gym as a personal trainer. I was fortunate to be working with so many skilled trainers whose brains I could constantly pick for different ways the body could be strengthened or trained. I was working on myself daily, releasing scar tissue, and realigning my muscular skeletal system using the energy techniques I had trained myself to do. The more I worked on myself, the more I became in tune with myself and with others.

One day my daughter injured her knee playing soccer. I took a gamble and tried my techniques on her. To my surprise, they worked. I saw and knew everything that changed or realigned as I worked on her. I didn't know how I knew, but what I knew was very strong and directed.

Eventually, this knowing caused conflict in my chosen career as a personal trainer. When I worked with clients, I could see the dysfunction and overcompensation in their muscles, and it made it very hard, ethically, to give them a workout program that I knew would cause more dysfunction in the end.

At this point, I took a time out. I took a job delivering Meals on Wheels for a while and the elderly clients were wonderful. I will never forget this one 85 year old woman, her name was Lillian. The second time I delivered her meal she started to talk to me.

She said, "What are you going to do for me?" I replied, "Deliver your meal." "No!" she shouted. "I can't get down the stairs anymore to walk my dog. My knee is bad, and the pain stops me from using the stairs. What are you going to do to fix it?" I looked at her in disbelief. "Nothing," I replied. "I'm here to deliver your meal." She laughed and said, "You know you can fix my knee. What are you waiting for?" We argued, and she looked me in the eyes and said, "God made you the way you are, so either fix my knee or don't come back." What could I say to that? She was up and down the stairs in a couple of weeks.

At that point, I was even more confused. How could she know what I could do to help her when I didn't even know myself? She taught me about intuition, about following your truth, and how – at any age – healing can occur if everything falls into place. Or, in her case, if she made it happen! During this time, word spread

13

and I started going house to house with a mat, doing whatever I felt directed to do.

Over time I created a full energy treatment which included being able to access the body and sense the imprint of old injuries and work with the client to help them energetically release these tissue restrictions. Then by using my exercise science degree, I work with the client on core strengthening, nutrition, stress relief to help them with overall healing.

As my story goes when it's time, what I need in life shows up. I was now working as a Healing Arts Practitioner using all the different tools I had acquired and then I received a phone call by a woman who owned a co-op of holistic practitioners. She felt I would be a good addition to her team.

It was amazing have the opportunity to work with Ellen and to learn from the other practitioners. Thank you, Ellen, for lighting my path.

As I continued to work with clients, my body was healing more rapidly, along with theirs. There is no end to the knowledge. Every day I still learn a little more about myself and how to help others. I also see in my clients that the longer they embrace the healing work (learning about themselves and tapping into the Body Within, their true healing potential, and energy cleaning as a practice), the clearer their life force energy becomes. Then they become more open to the endless possibilities around them – which allows them to heal themselves and, for some, others.

In this book, I share several case studies from more than 18 years working with clients to help them heal themselves physically, emotionally, and spiritually. As you read, use these real life stories to help you mirror yourself and how you heal. I believe if you take the time to really answer the questions I pose along the way, the answers will help you understand the depth from which true healing comes. We are all on this journey together to learn from each other, so happy learning and happy reading.

The Come and Go

By McKayla Jordan

Everyone has to come and we all have to go.
We come with a bang of joy and leave with a stream of
tears.
We come and get showered with gifts.
Then leave and get covered with flowers.
Though it's easier to accept then it is to give away.
In our hearts our loved ones will stay.
And as we say goodbye we will rise to our Lord.
We will pray and thank him and smile for we have
returned home.
Everyone has to come and we all have to go...

Chapter 1
The Awakening

Grace is my mother-in-law. She has four children. There are four of us in the hospital room, but one of her children is missing. As I look over at Grace she looks peaceful, she is in a very deep rest. I wonder, in my mind, "Does she know she's dying?" Sadness hangs in the air, but there's also a sense of relief that she's not going to suffer.

Once the cancer reached a critical point in her body and pain became commonplace, Grace just seemed to make a decision...she was ready to go. It's been one of the fastest, most challenging weeks of our lives. Why did it happen so fast? It seems as if she knew her fight was over, but we thought we would have more time. She didn't really seem all that sick.

Suddenly, everything just came to ahead. Now, here we are at the hospital. There are so many people – friends, extended family, and closest family, all here to comfort a woman who always comforted them. All of a sudden, we're alerted that she's starting to die. Friends quickly exit the room. Her children and I rush in. It was just like in the movies. A couple of deep breaths, and she was gone. It was beautiful!

The energy in the room stills, while the quiet sobs of Grace's two daughters create an ominous echo. My husband, Grace's youngest son, and I stand by, overwhelmed by the days leading to this moment. I am momentarily distracted as I realize her oldest son is not here. My heart sinks for Joe, knowing that he missed his final moment with the one person he loved and trusted most in life. How was he going to handle not saying goodbye? Less than a minute or two later, someone comes to the door and says Joe is on his way. He was in the lobby getting on the elevator. Now, everyone in the room realizes Joe is missing.

As I stand there, I start to feel the energy in the room change from very somber to a state in which I feel a strong energetic pull in my direction. It startles me. Then, a strange awareness comes over me. At that moment, I realize that Grace *knows I* am the fourth person in the room. In retrospect, it makes perfect sense.

Grace was not only my mother-in-law, she was always my biggest supporter of working with energy. She admitted that she didn't understand what it was, or how it worked, but she knew, deep down, that I was different, and this is what I should be doing.

As I settle into the energy shift in the room, I know what I need to do. I slowly walk back away from the bed. All eyes are on Grace as she lay lifeless in her just-passed energy. As I move to the corner of the room, I raise my hands and simply give energy to the scenario unfolding in front of me. My intuition tells me what's going to happen, but my brain says, "You're nuts! This can't happen." I just keep getting the feeling that all I need to do is hold space and be open; the rest will take care of itself.

About a minute or two pass; it seems like hours. Then it happens. Grace starts to breathe again. It's a little scary at first, but then she starts to breathe in a rhythm as if she's coming back to life. All eyes are fixed on Grace, wondering why this is happening.

The door opens. Joe runs in, grabs his mother's hand, and tells her he's here. As he holds her hand, her breathing becomes normal. Joe says to her, "Mom, I love you. It's okay to go," and again, just like in the movies, Grace does it a second time. A few short breaths, an exhale, and she's gone.

I'm still standing in the corner holding space, watching as if I were at a play. The mood around the bed is solemn. Meanwhile, I'm in the corner stunned, excited, happy, but also deeply saddened that she's actually gone. I start coming back to reality and try to process what just happened. The questions start racing through my mind. Why did Grace do this for her son? The answers come in a flood of awarenesses...experiences I've had with this family over the past 25 years. Grace knew that after Joe's dad died, his life was very challenging for years. She knew, of all her children, Joe was the one who needed to say good-bye, or he would struggle for a long time. It was her last act as a loving, devoted, matriarch of her family.

As I stand by in dismay, not having the slightest idea how to process any of it, I'm aware of all the different interactions in the room. Grace is gone, her children are consoling each another while I'm in the same room, but on the outside looking in.

As we all pitch in to pack up Grace's belongings before heading home, the children are focused on her dying and how life is going to be without her. Nothing is said, there's no discussion. At that point, I'm not sure myself what happened. The questions are flooding my mind. Did Grace die and then come back, just in time, to say goodbye to her eldest son? If she did, how? Should we all be able to die like that? I do my best quieting the questions for the next few days, trying to support everyone from the monumental loss we've all suffered. I knew, in time, it would all sort itself out.

Chapter 2
It Is What It Is

So, Why Grace? Why was she able to control her ending so beautifully?

Grace was one of the most realistic people I've ever met. She was a little too worrisome in life, which made it hard for people to see her in her true glory. She was an observer of life, and her life's choices brought her to her defining moment. For 15 years, Grace worked in housekeeping on the oncology floor of a hospital.

She not only cleaned patient rooms, but she talked with them, the nurses, and the doctors. She observed life at its most vulnerable for most, and she saw some of the good, and some of the most painful moments, for many. Grace followed a lot of patients and their struggles. She always knew, someday, it might be her own. She also knew that all her observations and life experience were going to show her how to help herself.

Grace had her own vision of how she wanted life to be. She knew if she got sick and was terminal, it didn't have to be painful. She knew death shouldn't be feared; it's part of life. We're all here for a certain amount of time, and in her wisdom, she understood that sometimes it's not about quantity, it's about quality.

You see, 12 years before Grace's story, her husband, John, died of colon cancer. In the end stages of his cancer, John's kidneys started to fail, and his doctors wanted to put a stent in to help drain them. Grace didn't want that because she knew, from all she had seen, that if he died from kidney failure, he would get a high fever, go into a coma, and die peacefully. Inserting a stent meant, yes, he would have more time with his family and yes, she would cherish it dearly but she knew John would probably die from the cancer, not kidney failure, and his death would be more drawn out and painful.

John and his doctors really felt more time was the better option, so they decided on putting in the stent. Grace was very disappointed he made that decision. She was happy for the extra time but she knew that, as difficult as it is, sometimes nature needs to take its course. From early on, Grace knew her truth about life and death.

After John chose his treatment, it was only a short time later that his ending was as she expected, not only for him, but for his family. When it was getting closer to her time, Grace took the opposite approach and wouldn't allow her doctors to do anything that would prolong her life to a point where she felt it was more about quantity than quality.

Grace knew, at an intuitive level inside herself, that death is as beautiful as birth. If we can understand that and fear it less, it can be an amazing exchange of wisdom and love for everyone involved.

Grace was an amazing teacher!

Medicine, society, and the drive for our last breath do not allow us to know when enough is enough. This is what I feel our ultimate journey is all about -- to be in touch with who you are, and to know *your* truth, so when making choices everyday in life, all the way until it is time to end your journey, the impossible is possible. The more we understand ourselves, love ourselves, and trust in the journey we're on, we, too, will know when enough is enough. I would like to take a moment and end this chapter with a toast to my mother in law – my friend and my teacher. Thank you!

Chapter 3
Mary

Mary is a 13 year old girl. Her mom takes her to the doctor for right sided abdominal pain. The doctor thinks her appendix is the problem, so he performs surgery. Unfortunately, it wasn't a correct diagnosis. While in surgery, the doctor explores her abdominal cavity, but he doesn't find anything to explain her symptoms. Next, he orders an upper GI, lower GI, colonoscopy, barium enema, etc. They still can't find the cause of Mary's pain. Bed rest is the only thing that seems to help. After three months of bed rest, multiple diagnostic tests, and home schooling, Mom and Mary still don't have answers. The treatment plan was to start Mary on nerve blocks at the pain center or go in, again, surgically to look around. Mom and Mary have already made a few trips to a large hospital in Boston, and this was the plan they came up with based on the information at hand.

I met mom and Mary at their home, and told them I would do my best to help. I took a complete history of previous injuries. Mary fell and split her head open four years prior, broke her fifth rib two years prior on the right side, and twisted her right knee six months before pain onset. I watched Mary in her bed, curled up like a ball, and as soon as she straightened her body, the pain flared up.

As I tapped into Mary's energy, I could sense the pain was coming from what some practitioners call myofascial pain syndrome. Myofascial pain is caused by the misalignment of fascia surrounding the muscles. When muscles atrophy from lack of use, the tissue around the muscle shrinks and twists. Getting up and moving the area (exercise) helps increase the blood flow to the muscles and strengthens them to pull the fascia straight. Sometimes it works itself out easily, but in Mary's case, her sedentary lifestyle, the extra injuries and now surgical scar tissue made the fascia twist and adhere to different parts of the body.

When muscles sustain injury to their fibers, the surrounding fascia shortens and tightens in response to the injury. Unequal muscle tension can cause compression of both nerves and muscles, resulting in pain. In a lot of ways, it's considered phantom pain. There's no reason for the pain, but the pain is really there.

Thankfully, there is a lot of research currently being done to prove, scientifically, how fascia affects the body from a rehabilitation standpoint. Last year in British Columbia the fascia research congress held a conference as a collaboration of clinicians and scientists sharing and learning to progress the field of fascia research. To find out more go to FasciaCongress.org.

If we look at Mary's past injuries, they were all to the right side of her body. Her lifestyle was sedentary, and she was house bound and overweight. Physically, her muscles were weak to begin with, and there was no stability in her core to hold her spine upright. This caused the muscles to weaken and the fascia and scar tissue to twist. A strong core and spine keep you upright and erect, whereas a weak one will not allow that. Look around at society – your peers, coworkers, family – and you'll see how sedentary lifestyles and work environments contribute to the problem. Especially troubling are the children who spend countless hours on computers and video games instead of engaging in physical activity such as sports and outdoor play. This does not bode well for their future health.

After energetically assessing Mary, I was able to pinpoint exactly what I felt was going on. From there, I did my good practitioner duty. I said to mom, "There's a good chance this is myofascial pain syndrome. I know a physical therapist with excellent credentials and experience in this area. You should take Mary to see her for an evaluation. " Mom was excited there might be an answer, after all. Mom talked to the doctors and gave them all the information. They refused to send Mary to a physical therapist. They said the information I provided wasn't an adequate diagnosis, and that mom should proceed with the specialist's recommendations. Mom tried to present her case again, but there was no support.

Mom decided to bring Mary in to see if I could help. In one visit, Mary was walking upright. In four visits, she was pain free. Then, the hard part began. Because Mary was in bed for three months, her weak muscle tone, bone loss and weight gain made her a *must* for physical therapy, but the doctors wouldn't send her to a physical therapist. They felt the problem was resolved without Western medical intervention, so Mary must have been faking! Mom and daughter would have to do this on their own. At that point, they were overwhelmed and bewildered because Western medicine was not able to help them. Mary found pain relief and a direction with my work, but because she did not go the Western route, there was no support for her care.

As much as I explained why the energy treatment helped, mom and Mary didn't completely understand. They tried to educate themselves about weak muscle tone and why the risk for re-injury was so high. Lack of knowledge and support from a familiar place – their doctors – made the situation even more difficult. It was definitely myofascial twisting. However, the condition was so foreign to them and using energy to help resolve it just didn't make sense, they only cared that the pain was gone and now Mary could get back to her life. As weak as she was, and lying down for much of the previous three months, Mary was prone to continued myofascial twisting and injury.

In other words, without strengthening, Mary was an accident waiting to happen. I did the best I could. I provided information, but the rest was up to them. We had our ups and downs, but eventually Mary was doing really well. I hadn't seen them for six months when mom brought Mary back to see me. According to mom, Mary's had a severe headache since her tonsils were removed a month ago. Considering her past history, I strongly suspected that the tissue and fascia around Mary's cervical vertebrae and shoulders became twisted during surgery. I suggested to mom that she should get a referral to a chiropractor or an osteopath. Either would be a perfect match. Just like MD's, an Osteopath (Doctor of Osteopathic medicine) completes four years of medical school and can practice in any specialty. In addition, they receive 300 - 500 hours in the study of osteopathic manipulative treatment and the body's musculoskeletal system. I gave mom names for both, so she would have more information to bring to her doctor. Surely, this was something Mary's doctors would be very familiar with and should be able to help.

Unfortunately, once again there was no support for Mary and her mom. The recommendations were not within the scope of what Western medicine would consider a proven treatment. So, what was Mary's mom to do? Mom had changed their primary care at this point and the same outcome prevailed. Once again, mom is at a complete loss. She brought Mary back to see me, to work with the energy treatment, and in one visit the pain was less than half. A few more visits and Mary was pain free -- for now. Once again, I counseled them on myofascial twisting and stressed the need for Mary to lose weight and strengthen, or she was prone to future injuries. If you're wondering why mom didn't just have me treat her, it's because I'm self pay. My work is intuitive and facilitated with energy and the help of the patient. Hence, it is not covered by insurance. Understandably, Mom didn't want to spend money out of pocket if she could get support from her doctors and insurance to pay. I totally respect that and always encourage my clients to use that avenue first. We pay for health insurance to cover these costs. We should try to use it when we can.

Mary did really well for a year and a half, and then she and mom were back on my door step. This time it was a severe migraine that had been going on for three weeks. She was on the latest and greatest of pain medications with no relief. Mary was now fifteen. I took another lifestyle history, and two weeks before the headaches started, Mary started kick boxing classes. Mind you, she was not very active prior to this. Is the bell going off in your head too? Weak body. Aggressive exercise. I energetically scanned Mary's back, neck, and shoulder area and I could sense the muscles were very tight and spasmed. When your muscles are strained and over worked, they create inflammation. This creates tightness in the muscles, nerves, and surrounding tissue areas. Could this be the cause of a long standing headache?

I asked mom if the doctors checked the muscles in Mary's neck and shoulders. "No," she said. "The doctor said it was migraines, so it's neurological." Then I asked Mary if she knew her neck and shoulders were that tight and she replied, "Yes." So, I asked Mary why she didn't tell the doctor, and she responded, "They said it was migraines so it didn't matter." Would it have made a difference to the doctor? To some, it should, but we'll never know. If you study anatomy, you know that the nerves run along, or in, the muscles. If the muscles are tight, the nerves must be also. There are different types of nerve pain, but this was definitely muscular.

29

We addressed the problem with the same course of energy treatment, and Mary's headaches improved with one to two more energy sessions. Again, I counseled them on stretching and strengthening, and suggested yoga or Pilates, and walking, until Mary was stronger.

Now, let's look at Mary's situation more closely. Is there a right or wrong party? Well, it must be the doctors, right? Or, wrong? You tell me. All the doctors treated Mary with the information available to them. The primary care doctor was at a loss, so he sent her to a surgeon. The surgeon found nothing, so he referred her to a gastroenterologist. He found nothing, based on his area of knowledge, so he sent her to a neurologist. The neurologist couldn't find anything, so that must be it. Mary wasn't experiencing pain in her knee, foot, hip, rib or anywhere that would cause her to be sent to an orthopedist. Even then, would he have found anything to explain her pain?

Myofascial pain syndrome is relatively new to Western medicine, but some physical therapists, massage therapists and osteopaths are trained to work with it to help manage pain. It's a real medical condition, and when these practitioners encounter patients who have it, they're able to achieve good results. The doctor exhausted all his resources, but then mom came to him with new information to consider. Shouldn't he have acted on it, or at least explored a little further? Each time mom went back to the doctor, he should not have dismissed the information just because he didn't believe it. If the doctor had taken the time to do a little

30

research, he would have discovered that myofascial pain was a possibility, and there are other modalities in Western medicine he could have used. Why didn't he?

What about mom? What's her role in this medical maze? Perhaps, she should have changed primary care doctors again and again until she found one who was willing to listen. Is insurance set up for us to do that? She tried once and failed. What's the cost to continue to change doctors and what are the insurance hassles? At what point do you start to feel the doctor must be right, and you must be wrong, especially when there is no validation for what your gut is telling you? Knowing what happened the first time with the belly pain, didn't that give mom more information to handle the second and third times? Should mom have done some reading to learn how to prevent her daughter from being in this situation over and over? Or, maybe mom should have helped Mary understand that her lifestyle needed to change? That she needed better nutrition and exercise after being sick so many times for so long? Shouldn't this have been mom's priority? Then again, how was mom to know it should be her priority if the doctors said it had nothing to do with Mary's illnesses? Finally, if mom convinced Mary to change her lifestyle, would mom have had to change hers as well?

What about Mary? Sure, she's a teenager, but shouldn't she have stood up for herself, and taken some responsibility for the third time when her shoulders and neck were very tight? She told me that she thought her headaches might be coming from that area, but since the doctor was so confident it was migraines, she didn't mention it. Why didn't Mary think her opinion mattered? Should someone have taught her that her opinion mattered?

How could things have gone differently for Mary and mom? I wish I could say that one party was wrong, and the others were right, but I can't. What I can say is that everyone involved -- the doctors, mom, and Mary – used the information they had available until more possibilities came their way. However, once there were more avenues to explore, why did all three of them shut them down?

As a society, we live in reaction mode. Your beliefs, fears, current knowledge, and wants come first before logic ever sees the light of day. When someone tries to tell you something, does reaction mode activate and prevent you from processing new information? We all do it. That's right. I said, "We *all* do it." When mom gave the doctor information that was unfamiliar to him, he drew back to his roots and shut it down. That's reaction. Had he listened and been a bit curious, he would have seen the bigger picture. Mom and Mary did the same thing with the doctors. The doctor said "No," so instead of insisting that he look further, or even insisting on the referral (which is something you can do with your doctor), mom reacted and retreated. It never occurred to her to challenge the doctor because that's not what she was taught.

If mom and the doctor weren't in reaction mode, each could have heard what the other said and maybe, just maybe, a different outcome would have unfolded. The doctors tapped all their resources, but then new information came their way. What happened? That's when what the practitioners believe comes forward. Once they go through the available science and treatments, you'll get what the practitioner *believes*. Then, you need to look at your healthcare provider. What do you really know about what they think outside of alternative or Western medicine? Do they practice what they preach? Eat right, exercise and get enough rest? Do they think it matters? Do you? Do they beat their family or drink heavily after work? I know that's extreme, but just remember when doctors, naturopaths, nurse practitioners, acupuncturists, etc., exhaust their usual medical protocols, you're getting their opinion. Just remember to ask yourself, "How well do I really know them?"

I'm fortunate to live close to Dartmouth Hitchcock Medical Center. It is a Western medical and teaching facility with some of the best doctors and science in the country. Every year, the hospital presents a community lecture series to teach the public about health. In 2001 the lecture series was called "Heal Thy Self." It was an eight-week series, and each week a topic was devoted to how patients can help themselves, in partnership with their doctor.

I'll never forget it. They put up a map of the United States, and it was labeled "lumpectomy vs. mastectomy." This was in reference to breast cancer treatments and how they compare across the country. The first slide illustrated that the science proved, in most cases, a lumpectomy was equally effective as a mastectomy surgery. After showing the science, they put up the percentage of surgeons who performed a lumpectomy instead of a mastectomy. It was only about 25 percent! This meant that women received full mastectomies, unnecessarily, when a lumpectomy would have been equally effective. The medical faculty presenters asked the audience if anyone knew why. That was the shocker! Even though the science proved that the lumpectomy was equally effective in most cases, the surgeon *felt* that the mastectomy was better. Their point was, "Do your homework!" Doctors read the science but, in the end, you'll get what they think and feel, not necessarily the facts.

The presenters of this particular lecture couldn't stress enough how important it is that a patient know the science too, and then make a decision based on what you feel is right for you. Sometimes, you'll think the same as the doctor. Other times, you'll disagree and do more research. But if you don't take the time to educate yourself, and just do what you're told, it may cost you an unnecessary surgery or treatments that could totally change your quality of life, or even end your life. It's your body; it's your choice. Make the choice because you know it's the right one for you, not because the doctor said so.

I want to help you develop and foster your intuition (what I consider the Body Within), so you will have keen awareness when this happens to you. I want you to be able to embrace new information, process it, and make a choice whether it's right for you –or not. Learning this now will make you stronger and more directed in your health choices. This not only serves you now, but it will serve you later as well.

Keep reading and process the questions of the next few chapters. In Chapter 6, I will give you energy tools to help you wake up the Body Within. As you wake up the Body Within, you will see how using it daily will help make these choices, and many more, to help you live a balanced, fulfilled life and open to creating a balanced peaceful ending when it is time.

Chapter 4
Sam

Sam was a 40 year-old male diagnosed with terminal liver cancer. I met him during the end stage of his illness and offered my services as an energy practitioner to help him with his passing. I visited him at his home where he was bedridden, unable to eat and severely jaundiced. I worked with his energy above his body and followed the guidance I was given. As I did this, I felt the direction very strongly and followed my intuition to clear his energy and work to create healing. It seemed like he was directing energy flow to his liver and creating health instead of working to pass on. I was puzzled. This is not what normally happens when someone is in this situation.

The next day, Sam called to tell me that he felt a lot better and was able to eat. He asked if I could come again. We did this a couple more times and then he asked if we could meet at my office. Every time I had worked with Sam, I went to his home where he was in bed, so I didn't know if he could make it up my office stairs. To my pleasant surprise, I opened my office door – at that time I was the second floor with no elevator - and there stood Sam with a big smile on his face. Remarkably, he made the trip himself and said he felt good. We continued our sessions and focused on the fact that his healing was coming from within. Sam was healing himself. We also talked about the importance of proper nutrition and rest, and how this would help prolong his time with his family.

Sam and I had worked together for about two months and things were going well. One day, he came in for his treatment, and his energy had taken a turn. He was no longer clearing his core flow, what I consider creating overall balance and health. Instead, he was taking healing energy into the belly area, mostly in the intestines. My first thought was that the cancer had progressed, and Sam had taken our sessions as far as he could. I asked him about this because it was such a dramatic difference since our last session. Sam admitted that he had started on a cancer detox program he read about online. The program was based on a popular book, and the website touted many testimonials, so it was considered reputable.

Sam explained that he was assigned a case worker that would help him with his treatments. This person was walking him through the protocol of drinking tinctures and then chasing them down with juice. This was quickly followed up with enemas to get the tincture out of his system because, apparently, it was somewhat toxic! Although it was toxic, it was supposed to rid his body of his cancer. I didn't know what to say. The case worker told Sam that he had been given a death sentence with his cancer diagnosis and this was his only hope to survive. They convinced Sam that this cancer detox program had worked many times, and they called him to offer comfort and encouragement during the detox process.

Shocking? Not really. You see, when Sam was diagnosed as terminally ill, he talked with his doctors about alternative options. They discouraged him and he said it made him feel lost and scared. Sam considered our healing work together to be alternative medicine (not a complement to medicine, which is what I consider myself) and since our sessions were giving him more time, Sam concluded that all alternative medicine must work. Hence, he refused to stop the detox program. I emphasized to Sam that I was complementary to medicine, a healing facilitator, and not all alternative medicines are reputable. Ultimately, I told Sam, "You are healing yourself." But Sam wouldn't, or couldn't, believe that. In my experience, this is the hardest concept for people to wrap their heads around -- that you really can heal yourself! Why do we feel we don't have the power to heal ourselves? Don't forget to ponder that question *Now* and at the end of the chapter.

As we continued our energy treatments, Sam would intermittently stop the detox program and begin to heal. However, it wasn't long before the case worker would persuade him to start up again. Once again, his energy would drop. It was a roller coaster ride watching Sam try to grasp the reality that he could be the one keeping his body going. He just couldn't trust that it was all him, so he continued to try more alternatives. He started using them simultaneously, with no real understanding of what they were or their effect on his body. He was living in reaction to his fear of death and, in turn, not making decisions that were beneficial to him.

Meanwhile, I watched Sam's personal battle with himself, and how his energy changed according to where his head was. One day, he was in control of his healing and his core flow was strong and focused. The next day, he was confused and giving in to everyone else. That's when his energy became weak and scattered. What's worse is Sam was in a lot of pain and the people from the detox program discouraged him from taking morphine because, in their words, "Once you went on morphine, you were done." Instead, they told him to take cayenne pepper drinks!

Sam's distraught wife watched in horror as he struggled with his own mortality. All she wanted was for Sam to be at peace and enjoy his remaining time with her and their children. Unfortunately, Sam was unable to come to peace with himself, and he pushed his family away. In the end, his death was lonely and painful.

Is this a rare occurrence? I'm saddened to say it's not. I have had many similar experiences in my work and they are becoming more common. Why does this happen? Can we do anything to stop it from happening to someone else?

Sam's doctors did everything humanly possible, within their scope of knowledge, to help him. But when Sam asked his doctors about alternative options, Sam said they discouraged him from using any modalities. They did not offer Sam any guidance. Yet, healing goes beyond what science has to offer. Doctors forget that desperate people do desperate things. Sam's doctors saw him as a patient who had run out of options that meant he had no more to offer. Sam saw himself as a person in distress. He just wanted some understanding and a little guidance. What if the doctor had seen Sam in the same light? Would there have been a different outcome?

I can happily say that all over the country there are cancer rehabilitation programs being set up in hospitals to help patients with counseling – pre-, during, and post treatments - diagnosis and treatments. The goal is to show patients things they can do to help themselves, and even support the patient after treatments are done. There are, at least, 100 or more programs nationwide. So, if you are diagnosed with cancer, search your area. You may be able to get the extra help Sam never did.

The other option is to look for a newer model of integrative medicine. There are many practices popping up all over the country. They have a board certified general practitioner, along with certified naturopaths, chiropractors, acupuncturists, etc. all under one roof, working together. This helps you get the best of Western and alternative medicine. The more we demand these programs and practices as a society, the more society will provide them for us.

As for the detox program and the case worker overseeing Sam's case, I am short on words to describe the misery this person created in Sam's life. He played on Sam's desperation and the saddest part is I am sure he truly believed he was giving Sam solid advice! I don't think such practices are an acceptable form of alternative medicine, but that's the problem. Without both modalities working together, it's very difficult for the consumer to really understand what is acceptable and what is not.

It bears repeating. Desperate people do desperate things. It's my, and others, contention that if doctors treated the whole person, not just the symptom or illness, they would see this with clarity. As for Sam's role in his own fate, I don't know. Is there a way we can prepare ourselves for a terminal diagnosis? Sam had to leave it up to his family to help guide him as best they could. Family can help, but if the patient is close minded and stubborn, they can only help so much. Some people handle their decisions well. They get very organized and map everything out. Others get depressed, go off the deep end, and make extreme choices. One thing's for certain. Sam was a victim of the people he relied on for help. He got different answers from his doctors, from alternative practitioners, and from his church. Furthermore, he wasn't in a good place inside himself *before* he was diagnosed with cancer. Therefore, he didn't have the balance to navigate all the information coming his way.

One of the many things I learned from Sam is one of the ways to help prepare ourselves for death, or a terminal diagnosis, is with childhood education in the home as well as in science class. We need to, not only, discuss the anatomy and physiology of the human body in grade schools, but also the natural process of death and dying and how it happens to all of us, sometimes naturally, sometimes illness, and sometimes tragically. Then maybe we might understand it a little better and fear it a little less. We leave all the questions about death to religion and churches, but it is a natural process that we will all succumb to one day and be exposed to at any given moment. Why is it the one thing we choose not to talk about?

Sam just wanted to live. But instead of navigating the process, Sam became a victim of it. He should have been focused on living and enjoying his family. I believe, in my heart, that if Sam had taken the time in his life to learn about himself and get acquainted with his Body Within, he would have had more tools to help himself. His intuition would have guided him instead of fear. That is the message I hope to convey, with the help of Grace and her story, and the many other stories I have for you.

I know Sam is now at peace. I hope writing this will give his struggle some meaning. I feel the best lesson we can learn from Sam's story is how to handle life. That is, how to be secure in who we are, so when adversity hits, we'll have confidence to make difficult decisions. If you can't make life decisions when you're healthy, how do you expect to make them when the chips are down? This leaves you at the mercy of others. Think about it. Who in your life do you really trust to help guide you in making the really tough decisions? Some of us are fortunate enough to have someone, but, sadly, many people do not.

This whole journey is about finding balance, intuition, and clarity. With that, we will be able to make solid life choices, career choices, healthcare choices, and maybe even choose when and how we die.

Chaos Breeds Chaos, Balance Brings Peace!

Let's all open ourselves to more balance and peace in our lives!

Chapter 5
Trusting My Intuition

There I was, sitting in the Intensive Care Unit waiting room with my family. The energy in the room was filled with confusion and utter disbelief. I looked around the room and wondered: Do I tell them? What do I tell them? How do I tell them? Do I really know anything at all?

Let's rewind to about ten weeks earlier. I was working in an office with several different types of holistic practitioners. The owner decided to bring in a psychic to join our co-op, and she asked that everyone get a reading, so they could refer clients to her.

Personally, I'd never been to a psychic. I really didn't understand what they did, or how they got their information. In my work, I try to empower people to know themselves and use their own intuition to help themselves heal. I'm also able to help clear their energy, so they can see more possibilities in their healing and in themselves. Sometimes I do know answers, but I like to think of them as possibilities.

This psychic thing was way out of my league. Nevertheless, I sat patiently as she shuffled her cards and made her predictions. I smirked when she said my brother and his wife were headed for a divorce, and there would be a fight over the child. She also told me I was going to need a household repair in a corner of my home. "It's a little expensive," she warned, "so prepare yourself." She went on to tell me a couple more things, including how I would relocate my office to a white house.

Then, she dropped a bomb. She told me my dad was going to become ill, be admitted to the hospital and get sent home. After being sent home, she said he was going to be rushed back a couple hours later, and he wouldn't survive! What could anyone say to that? My reaction was, "Yeah, right!" None of her predictions seemed plausible, so I just filed them in my memory and continued with life.

A week later, my brother called to say that he and his long-time girlfriend broke up, and they were fighting over the dog! (She was close.)

A couple weeks after that, I was on my hands and knees, cleaning a corner on the kitchen floor for the new refrigerator.

Then, quite unexpectedly, I found my own office space not far from my current one. I would now be working on the second floor of an old Victorian house. You guessed it. It was white! I gave each event a little nod, remembering what she said, but I really didn't think much about the rest of the reading.

Then, I got a phone call. My dad was in the ER. That evening, he was admitted to the hospital with a bleeding ulcer. At the time, I didn't make the connection. After about three days, the hospital released him. He was only home a few hours when my mom called to say he was in an ambulance being rushed back to the hospital. Only then, did I remember what the psychic said.

There we were, once again, gathered in the ER waiting room. The doctor said my dad had lost many pints of blood, and he was in a coma. He was being transferred to ICU to be stabilized for surgery, if they could do surgery at all. It did not look good.

I was stunned, not only because he was going to die but because she *said* he was going to die. I had a long talk with my closest brother, who's also very intuitive, and he agreed with the psychic! Now, I was confused and overwhelmed. How could she know this? How could my brother know? Why didn't I know? What do I do now? I did my best to comfort my mom, while my siblings assured her that dad was going to be fine. Should I prepare her? Say nothing? What should I do? I couldn't say he was going to be fine. I didn't know if I believed it. Yet, I didn't feel he was going to die either. I was just numb. I distanced myself and took a seat in the corner of the room. I screamed in my head, "What should I do?!"

It was as if someone in my head started talking to me, and I heard, "What would you do if you didn't know the outcome?" The voice kept repeating this question over and over until I understood. I smiled and thought, "I would do what I always do when someone's in trouble", which is sitting quietly and working on their energy remotely.

When I work on someone's energy remotely – whether they're in the next room or in the next state – I sit quietly and focus on their energy, or their Body Within. As soon as I feel a connection, I allow myself to be guided into doing whatever their

46

energy asks for. It is never the same for any two people. As I hold energetic space for them, their soul's energy uses the space to help them help themselves to create possibilities in their healing, similar to what happened with Grace.

Back in the ICU waiting room, I panicked at first, and thought,"If I start working on his energy, and feel him dying, then what?" "Well," I answered, "I guess I'll help him die." I had done it for strangers, why not him? I pulled myself together, found a quiet corner, and got to work. After about five minutes, I felt him working to ground his energy and heal the damaged areas in his stomach. I was shocked! He continued healing himself, and I felt he was going to be okay! I looked at my brother and said just that, "He's going to be okay." He just shook his head and thought I was crazy.

A little later, the doctor came in and said when they went in to stop the bleeding, it had already stopped. They re-cauterized the areas, and told us that if he made it through the night, he might have a chance. This was ten years ago. A couple more close calls, but my dad is still with us.

The take away from this story is that a lot of people look to psychics, mediums, etc. for answers. These individuals may very well be able to read the possibilities in your energy at the time you're sitting across from them. However, as soon as you get up and leave, you still have the power of choice. If you act based on what a psychic says, he or she will influence your journey, and ultimately, head you in the direction of their predictions. This will alter your journey's direction and limit the possibilities in your future choices.

It's all about choice. Make choices for your specific journey without the influence of others' beliefs. When you stop and think about it, how is a psychic any different from parents, teachers, clergy, or society who believe they know what is right for you? The question you need to ask is, "What do I truly know at a deeper level of myself? What is right for me, not anyone else?

This journey is about energy and growth. In order to grow your energy, you need to make choices that benefit you. If someone else gives you the outcome - you didn't choose it - you didn't actually remove any of the blueprints (learned behaviors) or negative energy from your space. When *you* make the choice, you empower yourself and your energy.

In this particular situation, I was creating a stronger connection to my Body Within, which was helping me to become more confident every day. As a result, I was able to put myself out there to help someone close to me. If I fed into the psychic's prediction, the outcome would have been negative for my dad, as well as for me, and my personal growth. What I want you to understand is that only *you* are the master of you! Only you can create the direction your life heads in.

Here's another story about a psychic and one of my clients, Sue. Sue was in her early 30's, professional job, loved traveling, nice clothes, jewelry, big city living, etc. Her family kept pressuring her to get married and have children. Sue didn't feel

48

this was right for her, but she wasn't confident enough to know she could choose *not* to marry and have kids. She figured it's just what you're *supposed* to do.

Sue went to a psychic. He told her she was going to meet Mr. Right in three months, and they would marry shortly thereafter. Sue was very excited, now her mom would leave her alone. When I saw her two months after the reading, she was getting very anxious about not meeting him yet. I cautioned Sue that it doesn't happen this way. "You need to be careful to not create it," I told her, "and just let life play out."

Well, at two months and three weeks, cupid struck. Sue was at a yoga class, the instructor smiled at her, and now it was love-at-first-sight. Ken was very spiritual and open to new experiences. However, he had very little financial means and was committed to his basic lifestyle. Sue: fancy, fast life; Ken: comfortable, simple existence. A match made in heaven?

Sue and Ken married about ten months after meeting. On their first wedding anniversary, Sue woke up from her created reality to see she had simplified her life, not because Ken asked her too, but because she thought she had to. Sue was independent and strong until her traditional blueprints came back to bite her in the tush! Now, she was working in the same job but had changed the rest of her life to her husband's beliefs, and the beliefs of her parents. Gone were the big house, fancy clothes, makeup and fun car. Sue realized how much she missed her old life, and how it really was who she was inside.

Fortunately, Ken truly was a spiritual person, and he only wanted for Sue what she wanted for herself. Eventually, Sue was able to move forward and claim her life back. It was Sue's lack of self-confidence that made her susceptible to the psychic's prediction. I'd like to think this experience taught Sue that it was okay to like her life, not the one her family felt was right.

These two very different psychic experiences have one thing in common. Both demonstrate just how dangerous it is for someone else to map out your future for you. I can't say this enough, so you're going to hear it again and again: Choices, choices, choices! They're ours, not someone else's. Failing to make a choice, you know you should, could cost you as little as traffic ticket, or, as you saw with me, it could have cost my dad his life and me my personal growth.

This is why tapping into the Body Within is so important. The more you connect with your intuition, you will have the confidence to make these choices without the need for someone else to tell you whether you are right or wrong. Your intuition is always there for you, you just have to find balance to hear it.

With that said, whenever anyone takes away your power of choice, it weakens your energy...it weakens you. Decide what you want, how you want it, and make things happen. Will it always be the *right* choice? If it teaches you something about yourself – whether you like something or not; whether you're good at something or not - then, yes, it's the right choice. As long as you're the one making the choice, it's always right. When the next decision comes along, you'll have tools, and a history, to guide you. There's no right or wrong answer; there's only learning who *you* are.

CHAPTER 6
HEALING AND ENERGY

What does total healing and keeping yourself in balance have to do with how things could have turned out differently for Sam and Mary? What about you and me? Is there anything we can do to actually prevent us from ever being in Sam and Mary's shoes? To answer that question, we need to delve deeper into how we heal. What is this ultimate journey we're on, and how do our decisions dictate whether or not we're living our lives to our full potential.

Why did Sam develop cancer? And why was Mary afflicted with all those health issues? Did they have a choice, or did these bad circumstances simply happen to them? Let's start with energy anatomy. I see us as a body, a mind, and a spirit. The body is our temple. The mind is the brains of the operation. The spirit or soul (what I call the Body Within) is the conscience, the part of us that is connected to the universe. What does any of this have to do with our health? Everything! I believe balancing all three is the key. We talked about balance earlier, but now we're going to learn *how* to balance, and what balance truly means to our quality of life.

If you have researched energy medicine then you've probably heard or read about yin and yang, chakras, meridians, outer layers and inner layers, etc. I really have no opinion on these spiritual theories. What I'm absolutely certain of, however, is that total healing is much more personal and goes deeper than we realize.

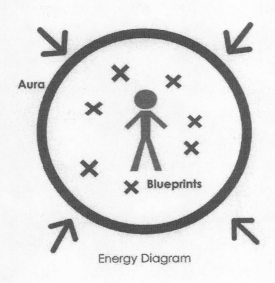

Energy Diagram

Let's start by looking at the diagram above. Imagine you're the person in the center. The circle of energy around you is your aura. Think of it as your own personal bubble. We've all felt other people's auras. Have you ever walked into a room and known someone was having a bad day even before they opened their mouth? You felt, or sensed, whether they were happy or sad just by standing next to them. That's their aura, or energy, hitting yours. Some people are better than others at reading people's energy or aura. Most husbands get grief because they're not very good at it. Moms tend to be really good at it. They have the ability to tell if something is wrong without being told.

If you're adept at reading someone's aura, it can be a very useful tool to warn you when to watch what you say. By the same token, it can also tell you if it's an optimal time to let it rip.

Inside your aura you have, what I refer to as, blueprints. (This is only my interpretation, it's an infinite universe.) We get these blueprints from our parents, teachers, society and even the energy you grow up in. They are passed down from their parents, society and so on. It's why you hate snakes and so does dad and grandma, but not one of you has ever met a snake to really have any opinion about it. These blueprints are behaviors, beliefs, food preferences, etc. Now, let's add into that space everything you've learned since you were born. That is, everything you were told about how life works.

This includes, but is not limited to, religion, politics, money attitudes, diet, even how to dress. Add in everything teachers, doctors, clergy, parents and others have taught you with since you came into this world. All these things make up what I call the muck or blueprints in your energy. Also, it's not just what they taught you; it's how you *interpreted* what they taught you. We all know how you can say one thing, pass it around a room, and everyone has a different interpretation.

This is especially true of children. How they hear – how they interpret - what we tell them. Here's a simple example of a child's interpretation and how it could have gone one way or the other. When my grandson was about three years old he loved the Wizard of Oz. Auntie gave Zack a pop-up book of all the characters and sat with him to look at the book.

She asked Zack who his favorite character was, and Zack said, "The witch." Auntie said, "Oh, you like Glinda, the good witch?" Zack replied, "No, I like the bad witch." Zack's mom and auntie then chimed in together. "Zack, you like Glinda, the good witch, right?" But Zack insisted he liked the bad witch. Mom and auntie continued to insist that Zack must be mistaken. That, in fact, he must really like the good witch.

I joined in and asked, "So Zack, you like the bad witch?" His eyes lit up. "Yes, Grammy, I like the bad witch." Mom and auntie rolled their eyes. "Why do you like the bad witch," I asked. Wide-eyed and excited, Zack exclaimed, "Cuz she's green!" Now, it was my turn to roll my eyes. If mom and auntie had convinced Zack that he really liked Glinda, would Zack have ended up hating bad witches, or perhaps the color green?

As children, how did we interpret what was said to us, and how do our own kids interpret what we tell them? We know what we mean, but does it match up with their interpretation? Kids will often just agree with what you say and come up with their own interpretation. Maybe a week, a month, a year or even ten years later, they figure out that their interpretation (the muck in their energy) was wrong all along. When that moment happens, their energy shifts and a blueprint dissolves. We call that an awakening.

Now look at the outside of your aura. That's all the information coming to you from the universe, or God, or Wakan Tankan, or Buddha, etc. (I'm not here to say which; that's your journey). That's your intuition. It's how you know someone needs something before they ask; how you know something is cancelled before you get the call; or how you know someone is sick before they get a diagnosis. We all know things but shouldn't. That is, there's no logical explanation for why we know certain things we do. But the truth is ...everything you need to know in life is all there waiting for you. But, how can that be if you can't hear it?

You can't hear it because your energy is filled with all the blueprints and muck you've acquired since childhood. Blueprints and muck are everything you *believe* to be true, not what really is. It's like shining a flashlight through a very thick, smoky room. The light is your intuition; the smoke is your muck. Hence, only a few rays of light can get through.

Now, I'm going to say something that may tick off a lot of New Age people. Having intuition does not make you a gifted person. Everyone has it. It does not make you a chosen one, and it certainly doesn't give you special powers above anyone else. What intuition does is help make you a balanced, healthy, aware, stress-free, happy person. Some people call themselves gifted when they know things others don't. It just means they're more open in some areas of their energy than others, not necessarily balanced. Here's why: Being balanced will help you to be open in all three areas – body, mind, spirit - not just one.

With my own healing, I find that every time I learn how to see situations in a new light, and learn to direct my thoughts and actions with more understanding, my energy gets a little lighter, and my body heals a little more. Plus, my intuition gets even stronger. There is no magic bullet! It's about you healing you, and waking up from your distorted reality. The clearer your reality, the clearer your energy. .

A big step in our awakening occurs when we become teenagers. This is when we start our journey. Parents, teachers, clergy, and others often dread these years. It's when we start to question what people have taught us, and ask ourselves, "Does it make sense?" This is when parents have a choice. Do you listen to your kids, even if it seems more like rebellion, or do you blow off their questions and opinions altogether because it's not what you think or believe? This is where intuition comes in.

The more productive, healthier approach is for parents to determine if their kids are being unrealistic in their new thinking. Or, could it be that mom and dad want their kids to follow the rules because they feel they're right. That's when parents should pause and ask themselves: "Do my rules make sense? Why am I asking this of them? Am I teaching my kids to think like me or think for themselves?" It's possible you're both off-track, and there's a different solution.

Here's an example. A client of mine, Laurie, came in one day and went on and on about her daughter, Sara, and how she wouldn't listen. Mom and dad tried and tried, but Sara kept making mistakes and wouldn't do what they said. I said to Laurie, "So, what you're saying is you want Sara to live her life the way you and your husband do because that's the way you're supposed to?" Laurie answered "Well, yes."

Then, I asked Laurie, "So, are you really happy with your life and the way it turned out?" She conceded "Well, no." Yet, Laurie still wanted her daughter to live the way she did. Who's the smarter one here? Is it Sara for trying to find a better way without help from mom and dad (and that's why she is making so many mistakes). Or mom, for trying to lead her daughter down the same path?

How do you think mom leading Sara down her path would work out? Isn't that when we become our parents? Isn't Sarah doing what she is supposed to do, making choices to try to figure out what's right for her? Why, as parents, do we think we know what's best for our kids? Do we think like them? Do they think like us? Do they have the same personality or talents? If not, then how can they make the same choices we make?

We all do it on some level. We have standards we live by, the key is to catch ourselves, to realize when it becomes less about a foundation and more about directing to what we feel is best for them. As soon as we become aware of our actions or our tunnel vision, we can choose to change it. As soon as we change it, we get rid of some of that muck in our energy and in theirs. The reward: More intuition and clarity come into our lives and those of our children and we heal ourselves in many ways. Sometimes emotionally, sometimes physically, and sometimes it helps us create balance to help us connect to our Body Within more clearly.

What is the most common culprit when it comes to blockages in your energy? Beliefs. Beliefs in religion, life style, even choices in medicine. Why? It's the fear that surrounds these issues. What if I question? What if I am wrong? Society has imposed such severe consequences if you choose to question these issues, it becomes a lot safer to hold on to your beliefs and fight them to the death.

We restrict ourselves with our fears and we don't even realize we're doing it. When someone asks you about these topics, or you hear or read something about religion, life style, or alternative vs. Western medicine, do you feel a defense wall immediately go up? Especially if it goes against what you know to be true? Before that wall goes up, maybe there is a split second of awareness when you say to yourself, "Gee, maybe I should question what I think to be true. Maybe, I should look into this further." At that moment, you *should* look into it further. Most times there is no awareness because these issues have been with us since birth. All the energy around them is, what I call, the foundation of who we are. If we rock the foundation then we have no strength. Think about when someone asks you about any of these issues, how do you feel?

If you feel defensive, ask yourself: "Why do I need to grasp on so tightly to my truth? If it's a truth, do you really need to hold on to it or is it just there? Are you defensive because you believe in your truth so strongly, you couldn't possibly be wrong? How can yours be right and all the other versions be wrong? Is that like hitting the Megabucks from birth? You were lucky enough to buy the winning ticket of knowledge! This is often the cause for blockages in someone's energy ... the internal struggle, the nagging question: "What if I'm wrong?"

The good news is that as soon as you have that split second of awareness and realize you might be wrong, it creates a little glimpse of light shining through. The purpose of this glimpse is to help you see more light. This, in turn, creates more space in your energy to help you hear more possibilities coming through. However, that does not mean it will change how you feel in these issues. What it will do is help you see if it is your truth or the truth of others that were imposed on you in your youth. Once it becomes your truth, it clears your energy. It's like this, if I go to the doctor's and he gives me medicine for my illness and I take it simply because he's the doctor and he knows better, then I create muck in my aura. If I go to the doctor's and discuss the medicine, question it, and take it because I feel it's what I need, according to all the information, a big piece of muck leaves your energy. Same answer, different energy behind it and you are stronger in who you are, having made the choice yourself not someone else making it for you. Who knew? All it takes is a moment to acknowledge the light, consider the new idea and things start to shift.

As we learn how we process information, we realize we use knowledge that we gain and spin it to keep us safe according to the weakness we have inside. That is what makes us create our own reality, rather than seeing reality around us.

I had a friend of a friend who claimed to be an enlightened being. He told me that I could never be enlightened unless I learned the way he learned, or learned from the people who taught him. I just smiled. What else could I say or do? Who said I was enlightened? Why did he think I was? Who said he was? In his reality, he was right and you could only learn from his way. In reality, it's a big universe with lots of teachers. How did he get so lucky to find the only one?

There are all kinds of reasons for energy blockages, some of them quite foolish. Here's a personal example, and one of my favorites. My husband and I ride motorcycles. Carl rides a Harley. I don't. When I first started riding, Carl told me the Rules of Riding and they are as follows:

The only real bike is a Harley. When we're out riding and anyone waves, they're waving at him – on the Harley. Harley people only wave to Harley people. (I call this the Harley religion.) Every time we go out with friends, the Harley riders gather to look at each other's bikes. No one even looks at mine because, well, it's not a Harley. They all have the same aura about them, and you're only supposed to dress and act a certain way when riding a Harley. Personally, I'm glad there are so many new bike builders to help these people open their vision a little --- and maybe expand their wardrobe a little too (wink, wink).

Now for the awakening. One day about ten years ago, my husband had no choice but to ride my bike. You'd think it was the worst thing that ever happened to him. I was on the back. As soon as he started to relax into the ride and enjoy it, I felt his energy shift. A Harley blueprint had just dissolved. Did he admit it? Maybe, a little. Carl's still a diehard Harley guy, but that day he realized there really are other decent bikes sharing the road! After that one little shift, he cleaned some muck and opened his energy to a new way of thinking. This led to more new experiences in other areas of Carl's life. That's how it works. One change can cause a domino effect of change. It's truly amazing once you experience it.

Now that I've explained how and why our energy becomes blocked, I'd like to share some tools to help you clear your energy and open your awareness to more possibilities. Some I have learned along the way, others I gained from intuition and guidance. I find each one to work in a different way so play with them and see if you connect to one or more, or even, intuitively, develop your own. Again, take notes as you read. If this information stirs up an experience or patterns in your own thoughts that you feel you need to work on, take a minute to jot them down.

As you experiment with these tools, choose one to work with at least once a day for a couple weeks. Give yourself time to process the technique and see if you can start to sense your own energy field. Remember, you're your own energy police, so take it seriously. The more you practice, the stronger you'll become.

62

Mala Beads

My first and favorite healing tool is mala beads. They are similar to rosary beads used in the Catholic Church. Mala beads are universal prayer beads that help you quiet your mind and train yourself to focus. You can move to each bead with a breath, a mantra, or just hold them while meditating. The challenge is to figure out what works for you.

You can purchase a strand of already-made mala beads on the internet or in gift shops. However, I recommend that you pick out your own beads and make the mala yourself, or ask someone to do it for you. This is what I suggest to my clients.

Why do I do this? Traditional ones are usually made of wooden beads, but I prefer the beads be made of stone, and you should select the stone that's right for you. Don't Google "stones" and just buy what you think might be a good fit. Someone else's opinion isn't better than what your own body can tell you! Instead, go to a bead or craft store and look at the display of 8 mm round beads. Before you pick up a strand, get a sense for how you feel inside. Feel yourself grounded to the earth. Then, pick up a bead and hold it. Decide how it makes you feel? Anxious, calm, tired, angry, peaceful? Do this until you find a bead that makes you feel peaceful inside. That's *your* bead!

A true mala is strung with 108 beads, but that's a lot of beads to hold. I suggest you buy 54 beads to make your strand, and go around twice. If you feel like you need to follow the rules, go ahead and make a mala with 108 beads! It's up to you! Choose something fun to make the tassel on the end of the strand. It can be cloth, feathers, more beads, etc.

If you choose beads for your tassel that are different from your mala beads, make sure they feel good together. Hold the beads together and see if it changes how you feel inside compared to how you felt when you held just your chosen beads. Make sure that, together, they make you feel peaceful. Then, bring your beads home, go online and find directions for making a mala, or ask someone who beads to make it for you.

Before you use your mala beads for the first time, you should clear the beads of anyone else's energy. Start by holding them in your left hand. Hold your right hand over them until you feel pressure, then scoop and throw the energy until you don't feel any pressure. The beads will feel lighter. Now, they're yours!

As you regularly use your mala, the stones will hold your spiritual energy. Keep your mala beads in a private place and don't let anyone else handle them. They are yours. As you use the mala, your energy will become stronger and so will the beads. Think of it as you at your best and clearest. When you're having a bad day, embrace them – hold them close to you and they will energize you, it will be you, at your best, healing you! That's my favorite part; it's your own backup of energy. But, remember, it only works if you use the beads regularly! A little note: You can clean the energy of your jewelry and other personal items in the way I explained to clean your beads.

Now that you have your mala beads, it's time to go on line and read some articles about how to use them. Don't just take my word for it -- learn, question, play, and figure out what works for you. If you want to recite a mantra as you go around the beads twice, I highly recommend the one below. If you don't have beads, you can still use the mantra by itself to help clear your energy. I have chosen this mantra for a couple of reasons. First, I gained it intuitively and it has been a core part of my healing physically, emotionally, and spiritually. Second, I have given it to many of my friends and clients and it has helped them achieve amazing results as well. Remember, this is only a recommendation, so if you see it differently, by all means, change it to personalize it for your own healing. Here's the mantra:

I am quieting my mind.
I am embracing my soul.
I am open to all possibilities in my healing.
I trust and have faith; I am protected.

I am quieting my mind: This means you are the power within yourself to quiet yourself!

I am embracing my soul: You are recognizing you have a deeper sense of who you are and are willing to tap into it (Body Within).

I am open to all possibilities in my healing: You are open to seeing all your self-imposed

limitations and their roots, no matter what they are.

I trust and have faith and I am protected: It means you are empowering yourself to believe in yourself and know that you are your own healer and protector. (No one else can be your protector of your Body Within; it comes from the internal power that lies in the Body Within.) You are your power. You are the Body Within.

The key to the mantra is to really mean it as you say it. Words are empty unless we empower them with our intent. See yourself seeing the words as you say them. Be careful not to use a specific intent with mantras. You may be asking for one thing but you need something else to create what you're asking for. Be open to what you need, not what you want or what you think you need. Again, if you see the process differently, then by all means, do it differently. Trust there's a reason you see using mala beads your way, and figure out what that reason is.

Quiet Sitting

If the mala beads aren't for you, try quiet sitting. I don't mean meditation, which can be toxic for some people. If you meditate and it works for you, keep it up. If you have tried it and struggle, try this. Find some place that makes you feel good and sit and observe. I like to sit and watch nature. Follow a bird, squirrel, even an ant – that's my favorite. Follow it, watch it, and figure out

66

where it goes. What do you think it looks like down in the hole? Or, watch bees collect pollen. It's easy; it helps quiet your mind and brings you peace, but mostly, it's about being present.

Simple energy clearing

If you're feeling overwhelmed, tired, or you feel like a cold is coming on, this is a great tool. Stand and put your hands at shoulder height. Push your hands slowly down the front of your body to the ground. Try to feel the resistance of the energy, or the air, however you want to perceive it. Do it again and again. It should feel easier each time. Your intent is to push the negative energy, that's on you, into the earth. You should feel lighter when you're done. Do this daily; it works well.

Solar plexus clearing

The solar plexus is located on your belly, just below your ribs. Again, whenever you're feeling overwhelmed, stressed, angry, just scoop the energy and throw it away. It may look silly, but works like a charm. When you're driving and feeling stressed simply scoop and throw. Scoop and throw. Don't feel embarrassed. No one can see you and you'll prevent road rage. Everyone wins!

Mini Me – Energy Clearing

Sit quietly in a chair. Put a teddy bear on your lap or use your mind to visualize a miniature (mini me) energetic you on your lap. Put both hands over the energetic you or the teddy bear. Close your eyes and ask for guidance. Just say in your mind, "Help me, help myself." Then, wait. You may feel nothing, you may feel pressure on your hands, or your hands may feel like moving. Let them. They may clear or scoop. Let them be guided and notice as you feel it in your hand, you may start to feel it in your body at the same time. Do this daily and you'll see how it gets stronger. Relax, don't try to be perfect. Just be with it and see what happens. If you can be patient and master this one, I find it to be one of the most powerful self-help healing tools.

Breathing

Another energy clearing tool is to work with your breathing. Just lay quiet, sit, or stand – whatever makes you happy - and take long breaths in, and long breaths out. On the in breath, bring in white healing light and on the out breath, exhale all the negativity in your energy. Use your mind with strong intent. It will surprise you when you feel lighter after the out breath. Play with it, do it quietly, going slower/faster, or at a normal pace. Most of all just have fun with it.

Light yoga

A lot of people find yoga relaxing, but it also can be physically stressful, especially if done improperly, or if your body has many limitations. The key to yoga is understanding the depth of it. Yoga, like most Eastern philosophies, is a practice. You practice every day, and you can always improve, but you never perfect it.

Yoga should be undertaken slowly and used as a way to not only stretch, but to learn total body awareness and presence in your body. If you find yoga comfortable and enjoyable, keep practicing and learning new poses. If yoga is difficult for you, find a good teacher who will approach it slowly and help you succeed. Try not to get frustrated and give up. It's really worth it.

Chi Gong

Chi Gong is an Eastern practice that promotes physical and emotional healing and balancing your energy. I like Chi Gong because it gives you a basic technique and you can build on it to make it yours. Like yoga, Chi Gong is a healing practice, never to be perfected only improved upon.

If you can find a master in your area, that's wonderful, but it's not necessary. Two good home programs I like are: Lee Holden and Ken Cohen. (www.leeholden.com & www.qigonghealing.com) Ken's is more traditional, Lee Holden is

69

for everyone. Both are excellent. You can read about both online and decide which one to try. Don't stress over which is right, just try one and learn. Remember, it's about feeling and experiencing your body and how it moves. It's not about how much you can do in a short period of time. Relax!

Nutrition

Nutrition is essential to balance and healing. I don't believe in diets but I do believe in listening to your body and eating what makes you feel healthy and energized. Fruits, veggies, nuts, complex carbs, protein. I won't elaborate on vegan, vegetarian, gluten free, etc. The point is there's no one diet that's right for everyone. Pay attention to what you eat, and how you feel after. If you are tired ½ hour after you eat, omit those foods and try different ones until you fell energized ½ hour after you eat. Pay attention, it really pays off. The body never lies, we only fool ourselves into thinking it is saying what we want.

Rest

Rest is extremely important. You should try to stick to a schedule, as much as possible, and you should never go to bed without taking some quiet time, to stretch and do some relaxation breathing. If you go to bed stressed, you will sleep stressed. Your body does 90% of its healing during rest. If your body is stressed, how can it heal? Again, you can decide if this doesn't work for you, and that's okay. It's all about choice. One choice defines the next choice, and that's how we find clarity in our direction.

Finally, I tell my clients that they should have a hobby. Ideally, these are activities that quiet your mind and distract you from the hustle and bustle of everyday life. Such as hiking, swimming, biking, reading, beading, crafts, fishing, etc. If you don't have one, keep looking and trying new things until you do. Your body, mind and spirit will love you for it!

Chapter 7
It's All About Choices!

I'm taking you back 18 years to a not-so-wise decision I made for myself after being in pain for many years. I chose to have a radical surgery to address thoracic outlet syndrome.

Thoracic Outlet Syndrome occurs when nerves between the clavicle and first rib become pinched. It's very painful and, depending on the severity, can really impact the functioning of the arm. My doctors felt it was congenital, that I was born with it. However, eventually I realized it had a lot to do with an accumulation of multiple injuries over time.

I had the surgery, and to put it mildly, my results were not good. I ended up with long thoracic nerve damage. I had a paralyzed serratus anterior muscle, which is the muscle that holds the scapula (part of the shoulder) to the body. The neurologist I was seeing told me it was a stretched nerve injury, and it would heal in a year or so.

Because of the previous injuries and the injury to the nerve in my shoulder, I had a lot of dysfunction in my upper torso and gait. My symptoms were severe headaches, chronic neck, shoulder, and back pain, and inability to hold posture, sit, or stand, for any length of time.

Three years after the surgery, I was still trying to get back to a normal life, but the pain and desperation were almost constant.

My primary care doctor sent me to a different neurologist, who did an EMG and informed me that there was no muscle; it never healed. Apparently, the nerve was severely damaged during the surgery. I guess I always knew because things weren't progressing as the doctors, physical therapists, etc. said they would.

My primary care doctor was shocked and upset. He didn't know what to do with me, so he sent me to see a top neurologist at Mass General Hospital in Boston. Mind you, I decided to go to appease my PCP because, three years after surgery, I knew there really wasn't a lot that could be done.

After spending an hour with the Mass General doctor, he told me, much to my surprise, that he didn't think my symptoms were related to the surgery at all. Nor did he believe the nerve was scarred or damaged.

No, my doctor had another theory. He believed I had a degenerative muscular disease called Wilson's disease, and he proceeded to give me all the gory details! Wilson's disease is caused by the body's inability to rid itself of copper. The body has a natural ability to detox most metals and toxins, but with Wilson's disease, the body just does not know how. My doctor figured all of this out by examining me for an hour, and not reading any of my surgery, neurology or physical therapy reports.

Naturally, my husband was devastated. I, on the other hand, was amused, and told my doctor that he was way off base. "Look," I said to him, "Three years ago, I went into the operating room with a different right arm than this one. I came out with a malfunctioning arm and right side of my body. I've been in this body for three years, watching some things worsen, and some things get better -- all while taking care of my three young children and going to school for my exercise science degree!"

I went on to say that I knew I was getting stronger every day, but the shoulder muscles just wouldn't cooperate. My doctor actually said to me, "You think you're getting better, but really you're in bad shape. Your body is really not that of a 35 year old woman. You have limited movement in how you walk and use your body. Your balance is off and your right side is almost useless. How can you possibly think you are okay?" I smiled and said, "You should have seen me two years ago. I'm so much better and improving every day." He just smiled at me, which I interpreted as a condescending smile.

Needless to say, my doctor and I had a heated discussion. He told me I needed to go for an MRI, a CT scan, blood work, etc. and see an ophthalmologist to determine if I had what's called a "Kayser-Fleischer ring," around my cornea. That is the telltale sign of Wilson's disease. I declined all tests.

At that point, my doctor and my overwhelmed husband were tag teaming, but I kept saying, "I'm the one in this body! I may have the issues you say, but if I have Wilson's disease I wouldn't be getting better." He smiled, and again insisted I only *thought* I was getting better. I explained to him how I had learned about body mechanics and myofascial twisting and how I was working on myself and my energy every day. I could see what the problems were. I just hadn't been able to fix them completely yet. I was here for help, not for a new diagnosis.

The shouting match ended with my doctor insisting, "This is very serious, and you're not listening to me." I responded that he was the one not listening to me! My husband, sitting there with a look of terror on his face, couldn't believe I was going toe to toe with this doctor. I knew he thought I should be listening to him, not fighting him. In the end, I agreed to go to the ophthalmologist. But, I told them, "I'm not doing any other tests unless I have this Kayser-Fleisher ring in my eye." They both relaxed and agreed, completely confident that they would be proven right.

Wait, the story gets better. Wilson's disease is rare. When I went to the ophthalmologist, I was in the exam room, and I could hear people in the hall talking about a "patient with a possible Kayser-Fleisher ring." I was practically in stitches because these medical professionals are waiting to witness this disease that I'm certain I don't have!

The eye doctor came in the room, and I said to him, "I hate to burst your bubble, and everyone waiting in the hall, but you're not going to find a Kayser-Fleisher ring." I told him the whole sordid tale to which he responded,"Well, your doctor is the best so, as much as you think you know, let us be the ones to decide what's going on with you. He then examined me, looked up, and put out his hand to shake mine. "Congratulations," he said. "You're right. You don't have Wilson's disease".

Now, can you imagine the upheaval my doctor at Mass General caused? For me? My husband? The eye doctor? Even the other medical professionals huddling outside the door? All because my doctor had credentials and I didn't. He said "Jump" and all these people did. I said he was wrong, but I had no voice until the eye exam proved it. What is wrong with this picture? Why didn't I have a voice?

Do any of us have a voice when we are with doctors, surgeons, physical therapists, massage therapists, naturopaths, homeopaths, chiropractors, etc? When do we know enough to help ourselves and when should the professionals acknowledge and respect what we know?

The hardest part of my work is showing people how to heal themselves. Even when they do accomplish this feat, they don't believe that they did it themselves. They blame me (as I call it), or a supplement, or a drug they took. Some also credit divine intervention. They can't grasp that they could possibly be their own answer. What has happened to us, as a society that we don't have the confidence to know who we are and what we're truly capable of? Do we do it to ourselves with the choices we make, or has society done it to us by making us think we can't possibly know our own healing potential?

I challenge you to make a choice to try the exercises from the previous chapter and find one that feels right to focus on your energy. Wake up the Body Within and get to know it. Then add in stretching for 15 minutes before bed. Do it slow and pay attention to what is tight and what is not. Then focus on the tight areas to see if you can improve them. Get to know your body. If you can't stretch in certain areas, use some oil and massage it. Get an anatomy book and see which direction the muscles go in and massage that way.

If you have had any injuries or have scars, massage and rub out any bumps on the scars and make them soft. You will notice the body stretching easier. You can even do it on your stomach.

If you choose to do the energy exercises, then stretch and massage tight areas before bed, you will relax and bring your focus on you – not the million things you have to get done. This will help you sleep better and help you heal while you are sleeping.

Next, I want you to really pay attention to what you eat and how it makes you feel. I also want you to learn about the nutritional value of what you eat. Make choices to change habits that are not serving you

This sounds like a lot, but compared to the amount of time in a day that you don't feel sharp, energized, and balanced, it's really only minutes of your day. The last thing I would like to do just before bed is to take a couple of cleansing breaths and ask your Body Within to show you what you need to see, and ask to be open to seeing it. This will help you to see the changes you need to make in order to create balance and healing.

What this will do for you is not only make you more aware of who you are, but you will know yourself better when you are faced with medical choices and someone else is telling you how you feel.

Don't ever give anyone the power to know you better than you know yourself. That's what healing is all about!

Chapter 8
Medicine

My work is complementary to medicine. I work with whatever type of medicine my clients choose for their healing. I try not to take sides on one modality versus another, but I am human, so I do have personal preferences. Here, I would like to touch upon both western philosophy and alternative philosophy. There are many other types of medicine, but in my day to day work, I work with my clients to try to help them navigate a system of Western and alternative medicine that are not always supportive of one another.

I really want people to understand that there is no right or wrong answer when choosing the type of medicine you need. There's only lack of understanding – lack of understanding about the roots of a particular medicine and how that form of medicine derives its answers. I want you to see that we distort how each one works, for our own personal agendas, rather than see the truth that lies behind both.

When using one modality or the other, you always need to be a major part of the healing process. The most important piece in any healing modality is showing you just how critical a role *YOU* play in your own healing. I am not sure either modality addresses that properly. Look back 150 years ago, and the meager tools we had available for healing in this country. How much did we have to help ourselves because of the limitations in medicine? If you didn't feel well, you *had* to rest. If you had an ailment, you sought advice from people you trusted. Then, you had to help yourself get better because the tools were so scant the common cold could, quite literally, kill you.

Now, we either go to the doctor, pharmacy, or alternative practitioner and get medications, supplements, etc. We read the label and take them accordingly. At what point do we even take a time out and ask our body what it needs? I bet most of us would hear the same answer. It might sound like, "Rest, less stress, better nutrition, more exercise, etc."

I find that people who favor alternative medicine complain about the overuse of prescriptions, and those who side with western medicine complain about the overuse of supplements. Alternative followers say, "Medicines can kill you, or damage the body. Plus, they only chase symptoms; they don't get rid of the cause."

Supporters of Western medicine fire back: "Alternative uses too many supplements and herbs that just chase symptoms too. They can interfere with medicines, but they don't have to tell you! They are not FDA approved so we don't know what's really in them. Who's right? Who's wrong?

What do you do if you want to try to use all the information out there but you are overwhelmed?

Let's look at Western medicine and how it works. Western medicine is mainstream, evidence based medicine. It's what most of us use our primary care doctors for. Then, if they can't help us, we see specialists in that particular field. This is what most insurance companies cover and feel is acceptable medicine. Its evidence based medicine. This means if 100 people break their arm, and they get put into a cast for six to eight weeks, 90 percent of patients will have the same or similar outcome. That's what makes for a proven treatment. Is it perfect for everyone? No. There's always an exception to the rule. If the first proven treatment doesn't work for you, you go to a specialist who brainstorms the problem and looks for additional proven treatments or drugs.

Are these treatments the only way to promote healing for an injury or illness? No, but they *are* tested treatments. Think about it. Any time your doctor writes a prescription, and you go to the pharmacy to pick it up, you receive a pamphlet outlining how it can help you, and how it can hurt you. The drug has been tested in a lab -- over and over again. This way you know what they're telling you has some validity. The testing and pharmaceutical companies back them up. Is it always 100% accurate? No, there are unforeseen problems with tested drugs; we regularly see this in the news.

That pamphlet you receive with your prescription details everything they've *seen* happen, but that doesn't mean other things can't. It's your choice to read the pamphlet, or not. It's your choice to use the drug, or not. And, it's your choice to *listen* to your body when you're on the drug to see how it affects you.

Where does alternative medicine get its treatments and how do they come to the conclusion that they work? First, you have to define alternative medicine. Alternative medicine is a range of medical therapies that are not regarded as orthodox by the medical profession. You can start with a naturopath, who has undergone eight years of schooling and training; to a homeopath; to an acupuncturist; to a chiropractor; to doctors and nurse practitioners who practice both Western and alternative medicine. Then, there are the people using computers to diagnose you with energy waves, or the practitioners who train in weekend seminars. Finally, there are the people who just say they're alternative medicine practitioners with seemingly no substantial knowledge or training in any particular modality.

How do we safely navigate such a broad system? Remember Sam? He just thought if one worked, they must all work.

Is alternative medicine tested in a lab over and over again to see if it creates a similar outcome? Again, based on my research, it really depends on who treats you. Naturopaths, chiropractors, and acupuncturists are becoming mainstream medicine and more accepted in the Western medicine circle because of their extensive training and their understanding of how to combine modalities. There is also more evidence to back up their modality.

Companies like Standard Process, Metagenics, and others spend a lot of money creating a lot of products and marketing them to chiropractors, doctors, nurse practitioners, and naturopaths, etc. They teach these practitioners how they're tested, how to use them, and why they work. They don't follow FDA guidelines because they are not prescription drugs. But, are these supplements used to treat and diagnose illness, and are they tested against the drugs from pharmaceutical companies? The answer to those questions is why there is a huge obstacle in merging the two modalities.

Supplement companies aren't required to follow the same guidelines as pharmaceutical companies, so it's hard to know what to use in conjunction with treatments you're already undergoing. While I find many supplements to be useful, being a critical thinker, I would like to see a label on them just like pharmaceuticals. I'd want to know the risks, benefits and possible drug interactions, or contraindications, so we could combine safely. This omission is why most doctors simply say, "Don't use it." They cannot prove it's safe and effective.

When I talk about the need for labels on supplements, all I read or hear is, "It costs too much money." Yet, the last article I read about the latest Cystic Fibrosis drug said it took one billion dollars - from start to finish – to get it to market. The pharmaceutical company had to pay that. If I were a supplement company, I would avoid that expense at all costs too.

However, therein lies the problem. Failing to hold supplement companies to the same standard as drug companies is preventing a genuine collaboration. Worse, it leaves a giant gap in the system for all of us trying to make informed choices.

My personal opinion is that specific supplements that are prescribed by doctors or alternative practitioners as medical treatments – in particular, for cancer - *should* be tested the same way pharmaceuticals are tested for cancer treatments. They should also be tested alongside the already approved drugs and treatment protocols available for cancer patients now. That way, patients are able to get the same type of information so they can make health care choices on a level field. I have so many cancer patients who want to take products such as probiotics, or green drinks and cancer specific supplements to boost their immune systems during treatment. Doctors and treatment facilities tell them not to, concerned that these products will diminish the effect of treatment. They don't *know* if they will; they just can't say if they will or won't. Meanwhile, the alternative practitioner says, "Take it. It won't interfere with chemo, etc." How do they know that, and the other guy doesn't? Again, who's right? Who's wrong?

Another big concern I have with how cancer is treated alternatively is the trail of evidence. I have many clients come to me who have exhausted all their time, energy, finances, and internal power trying to navigate a system that has no foundation, as I refer to it. If I receive a cancer diagnosis and choose the Western model for treatment, my primary care physician helps me to get to an oncologist. Then the oncologist sets up treatments and, if I don't agree, my primary care physician will help me find another opinion. There are also many facilities all over the country to help you with second opinions. Then you are able to find out more information to support what treatment is recommended by doctors, friends, or even the internet. If you have insurance, most consults and treatments are covered.

My experience with clients using the alternative model has been this – once you choose alternative medicine the primary care physician very rarely supports you. You have to find the practitioner or treatment center via word of mouth or internet search. There is no insurance coverage for your opinion, blood work, or treatments, so you are already in it for thousands of dollars. Then the supplements, IV's, etc. are all out-of-pocket, and most of your friends stop coming around due to the lack of societal support and beliefs. Sometimes the family supports the patient, sometimes not. There is no track record of any of these treatments, other than the individual practitioner showing you the evidence. It's very hard to find information online to back up this evidence. The second opinions are even harder because the next practitioner's treatment is completely different and costly, with no way to research it. That is why tapping into the Body Within and living in balance is so important to help you navigate an overwhelming system. It is also why progressive integrative medicine is vital, as well as places that mimic the Cancer Treatment Center of America model. It's lonely to have cancer, but it's even lonelier if you choose to use the alternative route.

We owe it to ourselves to be informed consumers when using either Western medicine or alternative medicine; I find the patient is usually misled into believing what the practitioner believes, not necessarily what the facts say. As I've said throughout this book, *do your homework.* Again, ask yourself: "How well do I know this person treating me?" Research your options, then...work on balancing yourself and listen to your Body Within.

One of the most prevalent misunderstandings I see in patients is when a new drug, supplement, or procedure comes out. Patients just assume every practitioner must be doing it or using it. They figure they don't have to do their own research because they think they'll automatically get the latest advances in medicine. Or, sometimes, the patient wants the new drug on the market, even though the old one has a better history. So, they force the hand of the practitioner to think their way.

Here's a perfect example. One of my clients decided to have a hip replacement. Betty did her due diligence, researched one procedure from the other and made an educated medical decision for herself. Betty chose a surgeon who practiced the newest procedure – he performed the surgery from the front of the hip. The rehabilitation with this approach is very short; you're up and around the same day or the next. Betty's outcome was very positive.

When Betty's dad heard how well the surgery went for her, he decided to have the much-needed procedure. But Arthur lives in another state. He came out of surgery with less favorable results than Betty, and a lot more rehabilitation. Why? Because Arthur's surgeon doesn't perform the new and improved surgery that

Betty's surgeon did on her. Arthur's surgeon still does the standard side incision surgery. You can imagine how stunned Betty and Arthur were to learn that the medical field still offers this older, less progressive procedure.

Arthur's two mistakes? First, he never asked his daughter exactly what type of hip replacement surgery she had. Second, he didn't ask his surgeon for any details about how he approached the surgery. Arthur just assumed, "The way Betty's surgery was done - - that must be how they do hip replacements now." It never occurred to him: "Gee. I live in a different state. I have a different doctor. I may get a different treatment." Arthur just assumed Betty had done all the leg work for him, and surgeries are better now, so it's his turn. Guess what? You get what your physician *believes* is right or what level of education the practitioner has progressed to or what the hospital he or she works for allows. That's not always what you want!

Here's another example. Many of my female clients have talked about using thermography for breast cancer detection. I was puzzled at first. They told me that thermoscans are a substitute for mammograms, and they're told its better at detection and a lot safer than a mammogram. The clients are claiming they are being encouraged to replace their mammogram with the thermoscan, that it's actually safer and more accurate. However, the company website actually states that a thermoscan should be used *alongside* a mammogram for the best possible outcome for detection and diagnosis, not replace it. Again, are you getting what the practitioner believes or what the science shows?

One of my favorite ways to learn more about navigating the overwhelming medical system is to listen to Doctor Radio. It's a radio show on the Sirius network. The show is based out of the NYU Langone Medical Center. There is a different modality on every hour or so, and their top doctors DJ the programs. They have a wide variety of guest speakers, from scientists to supportive medicine practitioners and individuals that write books on how to heal. They allow the audience, that would be you, to call in with your own questions about medical conditions, second opinions, or just your own advice to them. They help you understand drug therapies, the latest research, and the new and available treatments. My favorite part is how human the doctors are. Some of the DJs disagree with the guests theories, some DJs agree or are learning something new just like the listener. Some of the shows tend to be very conservative about mixing alternative medicine with Western medicine. Then with some of the shows like sports medicine and dermatology, you get a much broader view. Do yourself a favor and check it out. I truly believe it saves lives because of the information given, how it's delivered, and how they make you part of the learning. It's a great tool to help you make more informed decisions.

How are you making healthcare decisions? Are they based on fear, lack of research, or trusting in someone else's interpretation of the science? It's all about being in touch with your intuition, your Body Within, so when you are making medical decisions you are balanced enough to see the information clearly, not the way your emotions or others interpret it.

I met a woman recently who was a breast cancer survivor. Martha chose a mastectomy instead of a lumpectomy to avoid chemo or radiation. She also chose to have her ovaries removed to avoid taking hormone suppressors for the rest of her life. Martha did her research and decided these one-time surgeries would prevent drug damage, over time, to her body. She also knew the surgeries would rid her of cancer.

However, Martha then went on to tell me that she felt like maybe she had made her decision based on fear. "Maybe I should have tried to heal alternatively." I asked Martha why she didn't choose alternative at the time. Her answer? "My gut told me that I wouldn't be able to make the necessary changes. I didn't feel I was disciplined enough to devote the time and resources to alternative healing, I was not sure I knew a reason why I had cancer, so how could I heal it? I just didn't feel it was my answer."

How then, I asked her, could her decision have been fear-based if she saw it clearly, from all sides, and knew herself completely? She explained that since her cancer treatment, she had talked to her circle of peers and read articles about healing alternatively. It made her feel like she failed by not choosing that route. Let's recap. Martha did the research, questioned all sides, and knew her own truth. She then made a decision that gave her the best possible outcome. If that's failure, I would hate to see success! What I took from my conversation with Martha is that society doesn't reward us for bold, informed choices, so how can we really have confidence in ourselves to make them? So many questions, so little time!

Understand this: By the time you develop cancer, your body is tired. Furthermore, there's no true understanding of how you created it -- or you wouldn't have cancer in the first place. How long do you think it takes to learn the true depth of who you are? To realize that your genetics, family history, life style, environment, and choices you've made in life have brought you to this defining moment? If you know your truth, healing will prevail, whether you choose an alternative or a Western mode. Just don't think for a second that just the medicine is the real answer. The real answer, my friend, is you!

Medicine, whether it's conventional or alternative, has flaws. So, it's up to us to understand what our health issues are, to do our research, and when we decide on a treatment, determine the long term and short term effects of it. If any practitioner tells you that they have your answer, and there are no side effects to a particular treatment, consider those red flags. Run fast and hard to find a new practitioner! Any time you add medicine and/or supplements, or alter, the natural working of the human body, there is an effect. It's your choice whether you want to accept the degree of change to your body or not.

*You can create your own reality (*how you perceive the world around you and how you want it to be*) to make life what you* *want it to be. You can't create reality, (*what is really happening in the world around you*) reality just is.* With that said, repeat after me:

I am quieting my mind, embracing my soul.

I am open to all possibilities in my healing.

Chapter 9
Choosing Your Truth

As I peered around the corner and looked into the room, the hospital bed was at a slight incline and her hands are in prayer position. Wrapped in them is the rosary she's had since the beginning of her convent days. In so many ways, all the years spent devoted to God were very fulfilling for Carol. However, in other ways, Carol was a conflicted woman -- conflicted because she never fully understood why she had chosen this path for her life.

When Carol was a young woman, if you wanted more than to become a wife and a mother, you had few options, namely nurse, teacher, secretary, or nun. Financially, Carol's family was not able to help her pursue higher education, so she made the logical choice. Carol become a nun and devoted her life to the church. At first, her commitment to God sustained her.

However, as time went on, and the teachings changed, Carol started to see how the church was changing. She struggled with watching the personal agendas of those in charge take priority over the faith. Carol's own faith was shaken often over the years, and she sometimes had doubts about her calling. But after devoting so much of her life to being a nun – a servant of God – what else could she be? Who else could she be?

The years passed, and eventually Carol's fear of the unknown became greater than any doubts or questions she had about the religion or the church. She chose to shelter herself in what she knew to be safe.

Now, lying in bed, surrounded by her closest sisters, companions, and the little family she has left, Carol is at peace, knowing that the selfless life she's led, devoted to God, and the welfare of others, will guarantee her safe passage to Heaven. As she lies there still not knowing, or understanding, what it means to let go of your soul and release yourself to the next plane of existence, the fear diminishes as she knows her life of commitment allows her the opening for God, or his son, to come and greet her and help her to the next leg of her journey - Heaven.

As the minutes tick by, everyone waits and prays, prays and waits, and then…it happens. Carol's cancer-stricken body can no longer sustain life and she dies. Everyone in the room is saddened but also relieved - and confident - that Carol is with God now, her Father. After all, could there possibly be any other outcome?

Yes, there was. As I recount this story for you, Carol is still – as we say – Earthbound. She is choosing to *not* move forward because the forward is not what she expected. All her life she has given away her internal power. She has never truly tapped into her Body Within and had a true conversation with herself. She chose a life of others defining how she should think, act, and respond. In essence, how she should live. Am I saying if you become a nun, you don't go to Heaven? Absolutely not. The question I'm posing

93

is: When Carol chose this path for her life, did she do so because she felt it was her truth? Or, was it the truth she *thought* she had to live?

Many times over the years Carol questioned if being a nun was the right life for her. But she never allowed herself to make it about her, and what she truly wanted or believed. Instead, she allowed society, and what she was taught, to decide for her. Carol lived a life devoted to God, but was she living her truth?

Healing comes from being in touch with your soul – your Body Within, and understanding who you are and what you need to heal. Healing is about living your truth, not someone else's. If Carol never questioned whether or not she was living her truth, then how could she know who she was at a soul level? How could she be in touch with herself in order to free herself?

Carol's ending was surreal. The cancer, the seizures, the inability to care for herself, the pain and suffering. And, she wondered the entire time, "If I've done everything right then, why? I'm so young; I'm only in my 50's. Why?"

Carol and I have had many conversations since her death, and she is still in a state of dismay. All she has to do is move forward, but her reluctance to do so is reminiscent of how she lived her life. The safety and security of what she knows *right now* is easier than taking a leap of faith and trusting that's what's ahead is that amazing place she hoped for. It's just not the way she thought it would be.

Many times her gut spoke to her. She struggled with what she believed to be the truth, and she struggled with what *might* be her truth. If you look at how things turned out for her, was there peace in who she was, or constant unease in her gut? If she had questioned her path, she would have had to make some choices that might have diverted her from her chosen path. Then again, such a seeking may have led her right back to being a nun. This time with a doubt-free, absolute knowing that is who she truly was.

To be clear, Carol is not earthbound because she chose to be Catholic. Carol is earthbound because she allowed family, fear, society and the Church to decide her truth for her. In time, Carol will see that it is an infinite God and an infinite Universe, and no one has the absolute truth. That she has always been, and will always be, in control of her destiny. Is she stuck in limbo? Define stuck. She is where she is by choice or stubbornness. You can call that stuck. She wants what she believed to be true, not what is. How is that different than any one of us?

Chapter 10
Learning to Listen

My mom passed away from breast cancer and I thought I would share a little bit about her passing with you. When I tell people my mom had breast cancer they expect a story about a long battle and a tough fight. My mom fought for 31 days before she lost her battle with breast cancer. When we found out she had cancer it took them several days to pin point it to breast cancer. She fought as hard as she could to beat this horrible illness but unfortunately the cancer had spread through her body and she lost her fight 31 short days after entering the hospital for some routine "tests."

The reason I'm telling this story is if she had gone to the doctor for her annual checkup she would most likely be here. Her grandchildren would know her laugh, her smile and the warmth of her hug. She would've been here for the many "milestone" events that have happened in the last 6 years since she passed. Yes she is here in spirit and watching over us, we know, but it's not the same. I'm posting this because everyone deserves a chance to fight, my mom didn't get one. Early detection is SO important; it really is a fighting chance.

Kathleen White

What is intuition, or listening to your Body Within, and how can we use it every day to better our lives so we don't end up in the same boat as Sam, Mary and the nun, Sister Carol, in the last chapter?

What does intuition have to do with helping us heal or die peacefully? Better yet, how can intuition help us not get sick in the first place?! Let's start by looking at how often we ignore our intuition instead of embracing its power. On the following pages, I introduce you to a few people who either discarded or embraced their intuition and how living in a pattern of choosing one way or another influenced their journey. When it comes to intuition, you always have a choice: Listen or ignore.

My neighbor, Joe, passed out and ended up in the hospital. Many tests later, he found out he had colon cancer. Emergency surgery was performed to remove a large section of his intestines, and it was determined that the cancer had spread to his lymph nodes. Joe was very upset, and very surprised. He couldn't believe this happened to him.

Really? He was a smoker, drinker, and had never exercised or cared much about his diet. At what point, in the five years prior to passing out, did Joe not notice stomach discomfort, weakness, flu-like symptoms and, most of all, his intuition telling him something was wrong? Didn't Joe hear his gut telling him to go get himself checked? Furthermore, why didn't Joe go for his regular checkups? He was of diagnostic age to have a colonoscopy. He had a good job and good insurance. If Joe had done all these things, would it have made a difference?

Then there's my Aunt Lynn. She collapsed, went to the hospital and was diagnosed with Stage 4 breast cancer. She died about a month later. Like Joe, Lynn didn't go for regular exams or mammograms. Leading up to the day she collapsed, weren't there times when she just didn't feel well? Why couldn't her intuition get through to alert her that all was not well? She was a very intuitive person with her kids, her husband and her job. Why not herself? If she had been intuitive with herself, would that have made a difference? Her daughter, Kathleen, feels it would have made a difference. Kathleen posted the introduction to this chapter on Facebook in hopes it would make a difference for someone else's family. I hope it does as well.

Intuition is as simple as feeling the need to double check that you have your car keys, even though you typically don't forget them. It's feeling something is not quite right with a loved one. Most importantly, it's paying attention to the health signs coming from your own body. (This is why it is very important to be balanced and know yourself.) Listening to intuition gives you answers in all areas of your life - health, wealth, jobs, relationships, and your children. It helps you make better decisions for yourself and others. It could be little things like your intuition telling you to slow down. Stop taking on other people's drama. Relax more. Exercise. Eat better. Any of these sound familiar? Could actually paying attention to these intuitive messages be our answer to preventing our health crises, saving our marriage, getting along with our kids, or even avoiding adversity in our lives?

Our bodies are amazing healers all by themselves. If you cut yourself, your body stops the bleeding by clotting. If I cut off your arm, your body will immediately slow the blood flow to the arm so you don't bleed as quickly. How does it know how to do that, yet we don't think the body can heal other ailments and illnesses?

Intuition: (def) a natural ability or power that makes it possible to know something without any proof or evidence; a feeling that guides a person to act a certain way without fully understanding why

Everyday life is filled with moments to act on intuition. You get up in the morning, start to grab a donut and something inside says,"That's going to make me feel like crap. Plus, I don't need the calories. Maybe, I should take the time to eat something healthier. At that moment, you make a decision for better or worse. You start your day with a gut feeling. Did you ignore it or act on it? If you had acted on it, would it have made a difference in your day?

You go to work. Your co-worker, Sally, doesn't seem like herself today. Something's off. You ask if she's okay, and Sally says she's fine. Your intuition tells you differently, but you choose to ignore it rather than press Sally further. An hour later, all hell breaks loose because Sally was in a really bad place and snapped. What if you had just taken that extra second to say "Sally, are you sure you're okay? I have time. Let's get some coffee and just talk."

Every minute of every day is filled with these gut feelings. The most successful people in life learned early on to follow this intuition rather than get caught up in everyone else's opinions. The only problem is most of these people only listen to intuition in one area of their life, and feel it has no place elsewhere. I've seen very successful professionals – many of them clients - build impressive empires. They put enormous time, energy, and focus into their business with flawless intuition. Unbelievably, these same people have zero intuition when it comes to their health or family issues. It's not because it doesn't exist, it's just that they have tunnel vision.

I heard a statistic recently: 150,000 people die every year from drug reactions. What if we had a bad feeling that the doctor gave us the wrong prescription, or this medicine was going to cause us harm, and we researched it? What would the outcome be? That would be an interesting study. How many people have had that happen to them? I know many people, including myself who have caught a doctor's error. It doesn't mean you lose confidence in him or her, and have to find a new physician. It just means, 1) your doctor is human, and 2) ultimately, you're the one in charge of your own health care.

Let's reflect on Mary's case again. Wasn't there a point at which mom's gut told her that the doctors were wrong? Of course, there was. So, why did she continue to go back time and time again? Didn't she know her own truth? That she might actually know her daughter better than the doctor? But does society, and our medical system, allow for mom to know more?

And Mary … her intuition told her that the headaches might be coming from her shoulders but she didn't think for a second that her opinion had any value. Not with her doctor. Not with her mother. Why didn't the doctor or mom sense that Mary had input but was holding back? Again, does society, and our current medical model, teach that a teenager like Mary could possibly know her own body?

In fact, some teens do. I worked with a 17 year old athlete who had scoliosis and a lot of myofascial twisting. Kevin had high pain levels, and was looking for answers. We started working together, along with physical therapy, and he was getting excellent results. Kevin had to take a break from our sessions to go on a trip, and when he came back, it was time for a follow-up with his doctor. His doctor felt that physical therapy had not corrected enough of the problem, and Kevin's body had done as much healing as it could. Really? At seventeen, the body is finished healing? That really sucks if you're over twenty! In his doctor's opinion, the only option left was to put Kevin in a back brace.

Kevin couldn't believe what he was hearing. Not because his doctor suggested a brace, but because Kevin knew, in his gut, that he was healing and changing every day. He knew his body was moving better. He wasn't in as much pain, and he could reach and stretch in ways he hadn't been able to in some time. But his doctor was only using one guide to assess improvement, and he convinced mom that a brace was the medically appropriate next step. Kevin was adamant. In order for his body to heal, he needed full mobility and to continue challenging the muscles that hadn't functioned well. Kevin's intuition was screaming, "My doctor and mom are wrong. The brace is only going to make matters worse!" They thought Kevin was just a kid who didn't understand the magnitude of his decision. Let's look at this objectively: Kevin is 17, an athlete, and a straight A student going off to college. But he doesn't get a say in his own health care?

Kevin's gut was on fire, telling him that the doctor was wrong. If mom and doc are wrong, what can he do or say? Next time his gut talks really loudly, will Kevin listen? Fortunately, Kevin had a lot of moxie and his doctor and mom did what he wanted. Kevin continued healing and today he's at a good place, inside and out. He achieved healing no one thought possible. He was a very open young man, intuitive, and knew what was best for his health.

So, again, the question: Who was right? Was it his doctor and mom because they're older and more experienced? Or was it Kevin who was getting clear information from his gut that he was right? In this case, everyone was right. The doctor and mom made decisions based on the knowledge and information available to them within the parameters of medicine. Kevin used the information at his disposal as well – his intuition. But here's the disconnect: Kevin's intuition – the knowing coming from his gut – was not a proven medical treatment, so how could he possibly be right? Yet, look at his pain levels. They had decreased significantly. His spine was getting stronger, his range of motion was increasing, and he was finally able to return to his active lifestyle. Still, mom operating in fear mode, and the doctor, following medical protocol, decided that Kevin couldn't be accurate in his own self-assessment. Hence, Kevin wasn't heard. That is, until he pushed hard enough, and they finally listened.

Kevin was able to see reality clearer than most adults. His parents have done an incredible job raising him, now they need to realize the need to heal themselves. As Kevin gets stronger in self, his parents, who wanted him to see life clearly, now have to adjust to how he sees it.

I remember when I was growing up; there was an 85 year old woman who lived next door to us. She had married at age 14 and had her first child at fifteen, this was the norm at that time. When I was about 14 and just goofing around, she would yell at my mom that, "I was immature, and that I should be a responsible woman." She said I should be getting ready to start my family and learn more around the house.

In fact, in the state of New Hampshire, there is still a law on the books that says you can marry at age 14 with parental consent. I'm sure if any parents actually allowed their young teens to marry at 14 now, they would be severely criticized. In reality, today's offspring aren't considered grown up and able to make their own decisions until they're 21. They can even stay on their parent's health insurance until the age of 26. How many of them are able to make life choices and raise a family at 26? From a purely gut level, ask yourself, "Is this progression or regression?"

One of my favorite TV shows is NCIS. If you've seen it, you know that the main character, Agent Gibbs, always gets his man even when the clues or evidence say otherwise. His gut tells him differently and he keeps digging until he finds the truth.

So, here's my challenge: Take a walk on the wild side and go with your gut, even if it makes no sense. You may be right or you may be wrong. Even when you're wrong, it teaches you more about what you believed to be right. So, was it really wrong?

Chapter 11
Passing Peacefully

Here I am sitting in the neonatal intensive care unit of the Dartmouth Hitchcock Hospital with my three day old grandson, Zack, who had undergone life-saving surgery. The room was small, with just six cribs in the section we occupied. The crib next to Zack's was no more than eight feet away. Fortunately, we were mostly by ourselves except for the set of triplets nearby. It was impossible not to notice or overhear conversations as we were practically sitting on top of each other. It was apparent that one of the babies was very ill, and the doctors didn't feel he would survive.

The parents and grandparents were clustered around the babies, trying to process the possibility of losing one. I overheard them talking about the weak one. "I hope he can hold his own until the priest gets here," I heard them say. "He has to hold on." At that moment, I knew he was dying and they were hoping to get him baptized quickly, so his little soul would be protected and go to Heaven.

A short time later, the nurse said they were moving us to another area for a couple of hours so the baptism could take place. As we cleared out of the area, I glanced toward the very sick baby as I had been doing for a couple of days. This time, I saw the baby's energy detached from his body, waiting outside the crib, waiting to die. I was puzzled. Why was the baby's energy outside his body, not with it? Why not just die? Then, I remembered what the parents kept saying: "I hope he can hold on until the priest gets here."

Then I realized: The baby was reading his parents' intent. An hour later, we came back and learned that the baby had died just minutes after the baptism. My guess is that the parents' intent changed. They relaxed as soon as he was baptized, and the baby felt the freedom to let go. Would you consider this a peaceful dying? As soon as the baby was baptized he died. Did he/she do it on their own or was the passing influenced by others thoughts and beliefs? Do our thoughts and beliefs affect others in our life, of all ages, trying to die? How can I take such a precious moment and pick it apart? Why would I pick it apart? So many questions, so little time!

Let's take another look at my mother-in-law as an example of how we all should aspire to end this journey. Not the details of helping her son, but how she was able to do it. Was Grace blinded by other thoughts and beliefs or was she living her truth of what she understood life to be? She was open to all possibilities in her healing as was I. She took a leap of faith in that hospital room and hoped I would trust what was happening and just let it all unfold. For my part, I felt the energy pull and had no idea what would happen, but my gut said, "Go with it, and you'll see." Neither of us made a decision based on what we thought could happen, or feared could happen, we just allowed it to happen. That, my friends, is the hardest part to process and the hardest way to live.

I am an energy practitioner and I foster my intuition many hours a day, this is a big part of why I could feel, and understand, what she needed. There are always events leading up to those moments, but if we can't see the choices or openings coming our way, we may take the right turn instead of the left. In lieu of an amazing outcome, you end up with the only outcome possible as a result of the choices you made along the way. My goal is to teach you to slow down, to see the opening, and to let the miracle happen.

I have read stories written about primitive tribes who know when it's time to die. They give their belongings away, say good-bye, lay down and let go. They die a peaceful, conscious death. Are those stories true? Can that really happen? Why can't we do it as a culture? Why do we fight death and have no concept of what it means to let go? Do we even know we're fighting it? I have a client, Bill, whose mom was in her 90's, and she just wanted to die. He told me all the time, "She should just let go." He didn't know why she wouldn't.

So, I challenged him and said, "If I told you to die right now, how would you let go?" He got frustrated with me and said, "I don't know, you just let go!" He thought it was easier than it really is, even though he didn't know how himself. After countless conversations with me explaining to Bill that his mother had no idea how to die, and that it was fear and many other beliefs keeping her here, I think the bell finally went off in his head. I could see he finally understood that she did not know that she was in control.

Bill brought his mom home from the nursing home for a holiday dinner with his family. On the ride to his home, she opened up the conversation once more about how she was tired and just wanted to die. This time, instead of Bill ignoring the comment as he usually did, he took a walk on the wild side. He asked his mother what she thought would happen, and if she was afraid. They ended up having a nice chat and Bill was able to comfort her, he explained to her that it may not be what she thinks but to just relax and let go. This seemed to allay some of her fears. They both saw a new way of looking at an old problem.

Mom had a nice dinner with her family and when Bill was driving her back to the nursing home, she died in the car. Although it was outside his comfort zone, Bill had relaxed with her and guided by helping her make the transition to the next step of her journey. I was so happy for his mom, but most of all, for Bill. He opened a new window for more possibilities inside himself. Now, his life has opened to many more possibilities ahead of him. All it takes is a split second of awareness to create a new path for our lives to take. So, if what you're doing isn't working, give some air to a new thought. Miracles can happen if we make space for them.

When I do energy work with my clients, I teach them how to lay hands on themselves and clean their energy, just like this book is designed to show you. When I lay hands, they can usually feel the energy moving. Sometimes, they feel the tissue healing and the body re-align as I hold space, sometimes they don't! When they do feel it for the first time, it makes them uncomfortable ("What is it I'm feeling?"), but in time, they find a sense of peace and realize it's all them. My intent with clients is always to help them, help themselves. Some clients embrace the practice, learn, and really make changes towards healing.

Others feel uncomfortable if I'm not the one facilitating. Some clients really work to master their skills and heal themselves. Other clients try too hard and want a step-by-step guide to relax and feel their own energy. But there is no one-size-fits-all How To handbook! It's about learning who you are, and what works for you. It's following your Body Within.

As you do the exercises and learn to feel your energy, realize that *this* is the energy of your soul. When you tap into your soul, you're able to connect and be guided in your own healing. Healing comes in many packages. One of those packages is dying. So, if you're in tune to healing yourself while you're here, I believe it will be an automatic transfer to healing when it's time to die. If you see and hear the cues you need now to help you heal – be it rest, nutrition, stress relief, re-evaluating relationships or connecting with your Body Within - when your journey is done, I believe it will all transfer to that moment of peace.

The biggest disconnect in most healing modalities is not recognizing, not understanding, how much ability we really have to help ourselves and that dying is as healing to one as living. I just want people to use all the knowledge available to them whether it is Western medicine, alternative, etc. You just need to know what knowledge is truly right for you.

If you look at Eastern philosophy hundreds of years ago, yoga, tai chi and acupuncture were commonplace. You were taught at an early age to learn about your body and police it daily. If you felt your leg was too tight, your yoga practice would help you access and stretch yourself out. If your energy was off, your tai chi was able to bring you back into balance. And if you just didn't feel right (keep in mind, you knew what right was because you policed yourself daily) you would see your Chinese doctor who helped you bring your body back into balance.

My point is it was *you* who knew if something was off. You caught it early and corrected it. It didn't take 25 years of aches and pains to pile up until a serious illness developed. It never got to the point where you ended up so out of balance, it affects your everyday quality of life, and every treatment is a patch, not a fix. It all goes back to self-preservation - your body, mind, and spirit. There is only one you in this lifetime, treat you with respect.

Your body is your temple, not your dumpster. As you learn that you have an energetic being, your soul - the Body Within, that's when true transformation starts to happen. As you become more aware of the Body Within, you start to understand its needs and how you can affect your quality of life.

As you start to feel your energy, you'll be drawn to such practices such as energy clearing, or laying hands on body parts, or sitting quietly. Let your intuition guide you. Only you know what you're feeling and how you're being guided to help yourself. The more you practice, the stronger your guidance becomes. The more you listen to the Body Within, the more your life comes back into balance.

As you become more balanced, you start to realize what your body needs as far as rest, relaxation, nutrition, exercise, stimulation for the brain, human interaction, etc. Only then, will you really start to feel alive.

As you grow into who you truly are, at a soul level, you become one with your path or truth. All your choices become conscious, including how you live and how you die. You'll be guided because you know how and what you feel. If you've never tapped into your soul, how will you ever know what it feels like? If you don't know what it feels like, how will it guide you to what you need at the time of your death?

As a society, we're so good at keeping ourselves alive because we fear death so much. Hence, how could we possibly know when it's time to let go and how to do it? Do you really think those suffering in nursing homes really want to be there, or do they simply know no other way? Can we change that destiny for them? I believe some, yes. Some, no. Can you change it for yourself? I believe, yes! I've worked with many people trying to help themselves and/or their loved ones make the transition.

111

Over time, I have seen stories like Grace's become less rare. It all goes back to being open and hearing the messages coming from outside your aura. The more muck in your energy, the harder it is to see the answers when they're right in front of you.

Many clients and others have shared stories with me of their loved ones' final days. I heard two similar stories of people with young children who wouldn't accept their outcome and fought reality until the bitter end. They refused pain medication or anything that would limit their last moments with their children.

One ended up being admitted to the hospital and her young children couldn't go see her because it was just too painful for them to be a part of it. In the other situation, the children were in their teens so they tolerated it, but I don't imagine that they have a very healthy outlook on someone dying.

Death should not be feared, and it should not generate fear in those who witness it. Can death be tragic? Absolutely! Sudden violent death, death by accident, etc. But when it's a progression of life or prolonged illness, we should learn to become one with it and really try to learn that it's not the end. It's just a new beginning.

I've helped many people work with loved ones in the final stages of their lives. The more they opened the conversation to all possibilities – to help them see death for what is, not their fears, beliefs, or theories – the more peaceful their dying. They even seem to decide the timing. Fear is what keeps most of us here too long. Fear of the unknown. Fear of leaving family. Fear that there is nothing else. Fear that they weren't good enough, etc.

Back in Chapters 1, 2, and 4, I wrote about the passing journeys of Grace, her husband, John, and also Sam. My intent is to show you that, even in death, it still comes down to choices.

What do you think would have happened to that baby in the neonatal unit if mom and dad found peace for the baby inside themselves? Would the baby have stayed as long? How much fear of losing that baby was transferred to the remaining siblings? Will that be an issue, or blueprint, for them later in life? Peaceful dying transfers from one person to another, so does non-peaceful dying.

I was watching a news special featuring a doctor from Dartmouth Medical School who felt that, as a society, we've forgotten how to die. Doctors don't ever want to fail and the patient never wants to let go. It has become not only a financial nightmare, but it has turned us into an uncivilized society with pain and suffering that is unnecessary.

I hear stories from healthcare workers about families who focus on heroics for 90 year old family members – when it's really about their own fear of death. I've watched loved ones force heroics on terminally ill family members, even when the dying person just wanted to find peace. We really have to take a deep breath and learn about death in a healthy way.

If we're faced with someone dying, we need to ask ourselves, "What is my agenda? Is this really about them, or me? What do they need? Do they need to talk even though it upsets me

113

to talk about death? What can I really do to help?" It's all about taking each person and situation individually and really seeing that person for who they are and what they need, not imposing our own fears and beliefs on them.

As we wrap up this chapter, I urge you to practice the energy tools from Chapter 6. If you start to feel your energy flowing, keep working at it. If you have a question, visit my website and, hopefully, it will help you in your journey. The stronger you sense the energy, the clearer your muck becomes, and the more your intuition grows.

This will benefit you in all aspects of your life - health, wealth, family, relationships. And, yes, even when it's time to die. I wish you happy healing and a stronger connection to you.

Chapter 12
Childbirth

Natural Childbirth☐

Childbirth involving little or no use of drugs or anesthesia and usually involving a program in which the mother is psychologically and physically prepared for the birth process.

My niece, Jenna, whom I love dearly, was 8 ½ months pregnant. She looked about four months pregnant and was carrying the baby very high. Her partner came to me, worried that she might have a problem delivering. He felt it at a gut level and didn't know why. "I've always known things," he said to me, "and this is one of those times I feel something is not right."

I already had the same feeling, so I agreed to try and help mom understand. Jenna has a physical illness that's resulted in numerous surgeries on her throat and larynx. All of these surgeries and resulting scar tissue have caused a lot of myofascial twisting in her body. I suspected that the baby was jammed up under her ribs, and hadn't dropped anywhere near the birth canal.

I approached Jenna and asked how she felt about delivering the baby. She admitted that she was very anxious but was afraid to share her feelings. "Something's not right," she said. "I had a dream that I was delivering the baby and I couldn't breathe. The baby just wouldn't come out."

Jenna said she tried to talk to her OB about it, but she discounted her concerns as new mom worry! I wish I could say this kind of response was an anomaly, but I'm afraid it's not.

I said to Jenna: "I think someone is trying to show us the outcome can change. Otherwise, I don't feel all three of us would know." I brought her to my office and worked to free up the baby by energetically releasing the tissue restrictions in Jenna's torso. We worked together to release as much of the right hip and tissue restrictions as we could with the energy treatment.

As soon as her hip freed up her stomach started to dance. Mom and I laid hands on her belly as we felt the baby re-adjust and move down into position. We addressed the hip restriction energetically a couple more times before delivery. The good news: It was a short, joyous delivery with minimal pushing. The not-so-good news: We inadvertently proved to the doctor that it really was all new mom worry.

What do most people think of when they hear the term, natural childbirth? For some, is it simply synonymous with a vaginal delivery – but without drugs? Do women and their health care providers' understanding of natural childbirth even align with its true definition? What about all that pain and discomfort? Why do some women experience such unpleasantness and others don't? Do some just get lucky, or do they know something innately --

something other women have not tapped in to? So many questions, so little time.

I worked with Lisa who was 8 ½ months pregnant. We had been working together her entire pregnancy. Lisa had a myriad of physical issues, and pregnancy posed a significant challenge to her. I was able to help her during her pregnancy, while addressing issues as they came up. As I started our session on this particular day, I was struck by how different the baby's energy was compared to previous visits.

Typically, when I work on pregnant women, I only work with the mom's energy and I have no idea, energetically, that the baby is there. My understanding is, I help mom and it's mom's job to help the baby. On this day, as I worked with mom, all the energetic focus went to the baby's energy. Even more startling, the baby's energy was following the same rhythm and pattern as someone who is getting ready to die. At first, I was shaken. Was the baby in danger? I took a calming breath. Once I realized the baby's energy was shifting, it was readying itself to soon separate from mom for delivery, I relaxed into it.

When we're getting ready to die, our energy enters into a different vibration. On that day with Lisa, I learned that something similar occurs to a baby's energy when it's preparing for birth. And the best part? This awesome experience didn't end with Lisa. It's an energetic pattern I've observed many times with pregnant women I've worked with since Lisa.

As soon as I became aware of the baby's energy focus, the session changed. Lisa went into healing overdrive -- focusing her energy on healing some of the physical limitations that would hamper a safe delivery. There was an incredible shift of space in the abdominal cavity and a realignment of the hip area. Lisa's hips actually adjusted at that moment to allow the baby to drop into position right there on the table!

It's always amazing to experience the knowing the body has always had. Maybe, we just need a little help remembering. Was mom doing it or the baby? Probably, a little of both! In any case, Lisa's body knew what needed to happen. I had her focus on the baby and just hold space energetically. She moved and shifted her body with the direction the baby was giving. All I did was hold energetic space and watched it happen.

Over time, I've learned how to work with moms throughout their pregnancies to help them connect with their baby's energy in the womb. Doing so allows for mom and baby to work together to create the best possible outcome. I strive to make women a part of the process and try to teach them to work with the baby, not just the pain and contractions. When mom truly connects to her baby, an ongoing conversation is established.

For example, if the baby needs more space, mom is able to sense this, and accommodate. She can do some soft tissue work on herself by stretching and massaging, or even just adjust her body position to make herself and the baby work to accomplish what the baby needs for space. As delivery gets closer, mom is able to work with the baby to get in position and work with the baby through the labor. Some women have connected so well that their labor is relatively short, and with little pain and very little pushing. It's all about sitting quiet and listening to what's really going on.

Julie was another pregnant client who learned how to work with her energy and the energy of her baby. More importantly, she was able to intuitively read her body and prevent a potentially complicated delivery. It unfolded one day when she came in for a visit and told me that her left hip had a lot more tension than the right.

"It feels like the baby is pushing sideways into my pelvis," she explained. Julie said she had talked to her doctor about it, but he assured her it was normal pregnancy discomfort.

But Julie felt very strongly that this was not the case. How did she know? Did she really know, or was she just uncomfortable and assumed that's what was happening? My take? "It's her body. I'll take her word over anyone else's any day." As we worked together that session, it became apparent that Julie's intuition was right.

Together, we were able to get an energetic release in the hip area and as soon as the tissues restrictions were lifted, the baby started to readjust all by itself. Julie just sat quietly and watched her belly move as the baby moved into a better position.

I've seen this scenario play out with many pregnant women. The only difference is it's never the same restriction with each pregnancy. How can it be when no two of us have lived the same life or have the same genetics? Why do women have tissue restrictions that hamper normal delivery? Furthermore, why don't we consider tissue restrictions to be an issue? Would an obstetrician or midwife even know about them in the first place? So many questions, so little time!

Meet Karen. Karen suffered from severe scoliosis in the lower lumbar region. Her dad, a physician, understood the extent of her scoliosis and knew natural delivery was going to be a challenge. Karen and dad worked together to find a good obstetrician who would take all issues into account. They found a very reputable doctor at one of the best hospitals in Boston.

Surprisingly, this doctor didn't feel Karen would have any difficulties delivering naturally. Dad disagreed, but felt the doctor must know what's best. After all, it's her doctor's specialty, right? Karen was in the last month of her pregnancy and the baby was trying to drop down into the pelvis, but the baby ran into an obstacle.

Somehow, due to the pressure of the baby moving into position, it created a hairline fracture in her sacral area. This meant there was no flexibility in the pelvis or pubic bone, so her hips wouldn't open to allow safe passage. Still, her doctor wasn't alarmed. He chose to believe this development wouldn't impact a natural delivery.

Karen's attempt at a natural delivery didn't go well, and she ended up having an emergency C-section after many hours of trying. Fortunately, she and her baby girl fared well. Now it was time for rehab to follow up with Karen after her c-section. Unfortunately, rehab is not the normal course of treatment after a c-section. This hampered Karen's recovery, not only because it was a c-section, but because she had severe scoliosis.

Within three years of trying to regain her life back, her scoliosis degenerated quickly due to the weakness in her abs, and now it was so bad that her doctors wanted to surgically insert a metal rod along her spine to help support her spine. After working with her to help re-stabilize the lower ab muscles and strengthen her core, the scoliosis improved and so far Karen hasn't needed the surgery.

There has been a lot of research done looking at the weakness of the abdominal area and lower back after a c-section. Now, a lot of progressive hospitals and practices are sending women to physical therapy after a c-section to help them regain their prior lower back and abdominal strength. The biggest reason this has happened, like any change in medicine and in life, the awareness of yourself and what's happening to you and the knowing that you have choice, is the ultimate drive for change.

Why did I tell you Karen's story? Because there are so many important implications that obstetricians, midwives, doulas, etc. do *not* consider when it comes to the female anatomy. Women's bodies are not only being damaged by a C-section, but also by the extended amount of time spent pushing during so-called natural childbirth.

I realize one of the reasons there are so many more C-sections being performed is because of the long term bladder and uterine issues caused by excessive pushing. However, what really needs to happen is an understanding of *why* women are struggling to deliver naturally, and without complications.

My goal is to teach women total body awareness. If you know your body, and you're able to connect with your baby energetically, you can work as a team to create a more positive delivery.

When I meet a woman who's had a C-section because a vaginal delivery wasn't possible, I ask about the physical traumas she sustained when she was a child or young adult. Most times, lower body injuries such as broken legs, feet, badly sprained ankles, twisted knees or knee surgeries prevent the pelvis from separating at the time of delivery, especially if they happened early in life. This creates tissue restrictions up the legs and creates a rigid pelvis.

If you look at natural childbirth as it's perceived and practiced today, women are pushing for too long. The midwives, doulas, etc. don't give in until the woman is physically and/or emotionally spent – or the baby finally comes. Do the practitioners delivering babies have a real understanding of how little a women should have to push if "natural" is really "natural?"

My friend is an obstetrician/gynecologist and we were discussing deliveries. I told her how upsetting it was for me to hear stories of mom choosing natural delivery and ending up pushing two, three, and sometimes, four hours. I explained the trauma and side effects on mom's body and the trauma to the baby from pushing so hard against the pelvis. She said the medical community is aware of this; that's why they're opting for the C-section more. Apparently, a study looked at the long term damage to internal tissue, bladder, and uterus, from years of forceps, extensive pushing, etc. Now, a study is underway to determine if C-sections lessen the damage to women's bodies long term. I just want to go on record: Damage is damage – whether it's done surgically and clean, or from pushing extensively.

We need to learn *why* some women are having a hard time delivering naturally, the way the body's designed to do it, not just find another way around the issue. Society has tried to make natural childbirth the norm, the preferred method for delivery. But natural means so much more than what's currently happening in most vaginal births. It has to do with being completely present in your body, not only during delivery but during the pregnancy and also before you even begin to think of getting pregnant. It's about balance and intuition. Knowing you have the power to create the best outcome possible for you and your baby, not hoping you are taught by others to understand who you are and what you are feeling.

I talk about balance and clarity healing us now and helping us when it's time to die. The clarity in delivering your child is the child's first step into a balanced or chaotic life. You have the power, as a woman, to create balance in the first breath of your baby. How's that for an amazing start in life?

How we come into this world is the first step in our journey -- and it determines how clear our energy is. Babies are coming out of the womb with physical issues they shouldn't have, and this is how blockages and blueprints begin.

If I could speak directly to every woman considering having a baby, I would tell her: Get to know your body first; know yourself. Try yoga before becoming pregnant. If you find you have pretty good flexibility and range of motion, have at it! If you find yoga to be painful, and you've had many soft tissue injuries, look for someone in your area who does integrative manual therapy or keep up with the yoga and support it with massage to gain full flexibility again. This will help you access your body and determine if there are issues that can be addressed prior to pregnancy.

In addition, look for ways to learn intuitive energy healing you can practice yourself. The more in tune you become with yourself, versus someone else telling you what to do, the better the experience for you and your baby. You can start by trying some of the exercises I've outlined in this book.

If you're already pregnant and feel you have restrictions, look for a massage therapist that specializes in pregnancy to gain flexibility and range of motion. Understand what the process is, and really try to make the baby part of the process. Sit quietly. Put your hands on your belly, and focus on your baby. Ask him/her what they need and wait. You may feel compelled to massage certain tissue areas. Or, maybe stretch your hips or back, etc. You're not crazy! Your baby's energy will help you, to help him or her.

If you make this a regular practice throughout your pregnancy, you'll find yourself automatically adjusting your body position in the last trimester to accommodate and comfort both you and your baby. This will also tune you into the baby's energy so during labor you can do the same thing. You will know, without anyone coaching you, the best position to put your body in – even if it's not the norm for most women. Know your body. Know yourself. It will completely change, for the better, your pregnancy and your labor and delivery experience.

Chapter 13
How Do We View the World?

I watch people all the time and I'm amazed that we have no idea how our actions affect those around us. I was at a traffic intersection recently and an oncoming car had the red light. The distracted driver was on her cell phone, barreling into the intersection, and almost hit a car. The driver of the other car laid on his horn, and she finally stopped. But she never looked up, never interrupted her conversation, and never moved the phone in any way.

I don't know about you, but if I'm alerted to stop fast, I instinctively grab onto the wheel with both hands and hit the brakes. I think we call that – reaction. Where was her reaction? Why didn't she even flinch at the fact that she almost hurt herself and someone else? No matter who you are, I would think that close of a call deserved a moment of reflection. How could she not see the chaos she just caused?

I had another experience not too long ago that rocked my world, as they say. I was in my office working on a client, and I heard a loud bang. My secretary came running in and said that a car had just crash into a gas pump at the station across the street. The gas pump was toppled over and the car and the pump were on fire! I ran to the window just in time to see a Good Samaritan running to the car.

The car was on top of the pump and its entire right side and front end was in flames. The Good Samaritan pulled a five or six year old girl out of the back and the driver out of the front just before the car went up in flames. I was impressed at the clarity of the woman who saved them and selflessly put herself in harm's way. After watching this near death experience with my secretary and client, I was pretty shaken up.

We watched the car burn as spectators started to surround the scene. My office is about 200 yards away on the second floor, and I thought, "That's a pretty big fire coming out of a gas pump that shows no signs of going out." It was a very old gas station with free standing pumps and no overhead protection where you see all the sprinkler heads in the new stations. Nothing was happening to put out the fire.

I heard someone scream to the gas station attendant, "Shut the gas off! Shut the gas off!" But the fire continued to burn. Then my secretary and I had the same thought: "What if it explodes?" Curiously, my client seemed unfazed and didn't have the same concern. I got really nervous and thought maybe we should leave the building and move away from the scene. I looked out the window at the people still standing near the car. The car – on fire – on top of a gas pump. Was I the only one thinking this might be dangerous?

I grabbed my client and my secretary and ran downstairs to evacuate the building and move away from the area. It was a busy office and it was business as usual. I interrupted and said, "We

127

should leave the building, they can't put out the fire, we are all in danger." His reaction, and everyone else in the office, was unresponsive and looking at me as overreacting. I asked the owner if he thought the fire could ignite the tanks in the ground. His response: "Hmm, I hadn't thought of that." "Don't you think we are too close if something happens?" I asked him. "Nah, I don't think so" he said, and went back to working with his client. At that point, I asked myself if I was the crazy one and decided I wasn't.

Just then the fire department arrived. They quickly helped the station owner turn off the pumps and get the fire under control. The whole ordeal was over in about five minutes. I was emotionally spent and overwhelmed by what I had just witnessed. I thought of the little girl and how scary it must have been for her.

I sat for a moment then broke down. My client, on the other hand, was bewildered by the fact that I let it bother me so much. She couldn't understand why I was so upset and not able to just continue on with my day, that I just needed a moment to process it all.

Can we witness someone almost die before our eyes and not be affected? I watched my secretary, huddled at her desk, visibly shaking. I was shaking too, yet my client wasn't rattled at all. Why did the entire office downstairs continue with business as usual? We live in a pretty quiet city as far as anything like this happening. This was definitely an unusual occurrence. Why was there a different interpretation of the same experience? What about the people surrounding the car on fire on top of a gas pump? What's up with that?

We can apply the same question to other areas of life. Take politics, for example. What one politician thinks is important, two others don't. So how do we find balance in that? What about home life? How many times does the husband think something's important and the wife doesn't? Or, the parent and the child? Who's right? Who's wrong? That, my friends, is where the ability to view what is really happening, not what we interpret is happening, becomes critically important and life-changing.

I wish I could just write one sentence that answers the question, "How do we change how we view the world?" Unfortunately, I can't. The only thing I can do is to help you break down the barriers that cloud you from seeing what really is, not what you perceive or want it to be.

Why do so many of us want to see things other than as they really are? Let's look at another client, Barbara. Barbara was married to the same man for 25 years. They had their ups and downs. She would tell me about some of her friends and how their husbands were verbally abusive and controlling. "I'll never live that way," she said. "What's wrong with them?

After about two years of doing self-work, cleaning her energy and questioning why she and her friends saw the world the way they did, Barbara had an awakening. She awakened to the reality that she was in an extremely abusive relationship and hadn't seen it. Barbara had created her own reality – what she needed it to be – until she had the strength and tools to see it for what it really was. How's that for a bad dream? Now, what does she do? Most days, she wanted to go back to her bubble. Why? Once you become aware, you have to choose to make changes or live with the pain.

Let me clarify. Barbara chose her reality to protect herself. That's one reason for living in a created reality. But, it's not always about protection. Sometimes, it's fear, ignorance, belief that that's just how life works, or just plain stubbornness and an unwillingness to want to change. It's always easier to stay where you are instead of changing. Other times, it's the way you were taught – until you realize there are many other ways to see it.

Our distorted view of reality is what the Buddhists refer to as, "life is suffering". Basically, it says that only when you realize you're suffering can you see clearly enough to discover the root of the suffering. Once you discover the root, you have the power to change. But change can only occur if you see and understand the need to change. Healing is about taking off your blinders and seeing yourself completely. Only then can you live in reality. Once this happens, you have the power to create the life that truly makes you happy and at peace.

Here's another example of interpreting your own reality. Don was a seemingly healthy, 62 year-old man diagnosed with a terminal cancer. Don's family was very upset and just couldn't understand how this could happen. They couldn't believe how someone so healthy could get so sick, so fast -- out of nowhere.

130

Don came to my office and completed a standard intake form, which I read in disbelief. Don's medical history: He had prostate cancer and treatment, Type II diabetes, arthritis, heart disease, etc. So, *this* is what Don's family considered healthy? In their view, again, how they saw the situation, all of these health issues were treated, or Don was currently under a doctor's care for them, so they felt that meant he must be healthy. Really?

I have a relative who takes a similar view when it comes to her spouse's health. She called one day to tell me that her husband went to his doctor and they gave him a clean bill of health, "He's all healed up," she said. I scratched my head. Let's see ...he can't breathe very well, or walk any distance, he's tired all the time, and has a bad heart, etc. I'm glad he's so healthy! My relative interpreted the doctor's evaluation as "her husband's fine." I explained to her that, "He's as healthy as one can be in his condition." Her response: "You make issues where there are none. The doctor said he's healthy." What could I say to that?

When you only see what you want to see in each situation, you're helpless when things don't go as planned. My relative is always surprised when her spouse has an infection or ends up in the hospital. "How could this happen?" she asks. What kind of solution can you come up with if you don't want to see the problem? How can you fix something that's not right if you choose for it to not be there? There's nothing to fix if you can't see it, right? Oh! Then it's not your fault. You're just a victim of life!

Going back to Sam and Mary, how much of the distortion was because nobody really understood the situation clearly? Hence, the doctors and the patients made it what they wanted it to be which, ultimately, limited the possible outcomes. Just look around you. How do you view what you see? How do our children view the world?

Now that I'm a grandmother, I'm able to take the time to observe the parent-child relationship without being in it. I remember when my grandson, Zack, was about 12 months old, and his dad would be using his laptop. Zack would do a couple of things to get dad's attention, but dad wouldn't budge, so Zack would slap the keyboard. *That* would get dad's attention.

This became how Zack got dad's attention. So, how did this child know if that was good attention or bad attention? Is it because we tell them it's good or bad? Is there good attention and bad attention? Zack just wanted dad to notice him and he did. So, how does Zack now perceive his actions and when does his perception change? How will he get attention in school? With his peers?

The gist of it: We completely create how we view the world and how our children view the world.

I challenge you to really question how you are viewing the world. Do you see it like everyone else sees it? Do you have a different opinion on issues? Do your kids share your opinion because it's yours? Or is it theirs? Why do you see it different? Is there, maybe, a bit of distortion in how you see it? Keep asking yourself questions and observe your kids actions. I bet it's like looking in a mirror. The question is, is it a clean mirror or a mucky one?

As you start to see the world around you for what it is, not what you have chosen to see it as, this brings more balance and healing to your energy. As we bring more balance our intuition comes in clearer so we are more connected to our Body Within. As we live a life of balance and intuition, this not only serves us now, it will automatically transfer when we die. That, my friend, is a beautiful thing!

CHAOS BREEDS CHAOS,
BALANCE BRINGS PEACE.

Chapter 14
Creating Your Own Reality

"You can create your own reality to make life what you want it to be, but you can't create reality. Reality just is."

What does this really mean?

Let's take a look at some examples of how people can create their own realities.

Ten years ago, a close friend of mine was working full time at a retail store. She was planning to have her third hernia surgery in 18 months, and my intuition was in overdrive. I knew if she had another surgery so soon there would be a very bad outcome later in her life. I tried to make her understand the damage she was doing to her body, and how she really needed to take a step back to try and rectify the situation.

I kicked in to protective mode and went to her doctors appointments with her. I also got her husband involved to coordinate a treatment plan after surgery that would focus on core strengthening and stability training. I absolutely knew if she had this surgery and went right back to work she would not only get hurt again, but the long term consequences would be devastating. I knew in my gut that her bad habits and lack of respect for her body were going to catch up with her in a bad way. Still, I felt she had plenty of time to correct it.

The plan was for her to take four or five months off from work and do the rehabilitation her body desperately needed to heal. Her husband agreed, even though it would be costly due to lost wages and having to pay health insurance. The surgeon was on board, and my friend even had her own physiatrist (a doctor of physical therapy) in charge of her care. Everything was in place. She had the surgery and we were moving forward with the agreed upon plan.

That is, until my friend went to her four week post-op appointment and told the surgeon she was fine and ready to go back to work! She said she wasn't interested in the rehab program and, essentially, refused all help. What could the doctor do? He gave her a note and back to work she went. Of course, I was furious and didn't know how to handle it. My gut was on fire and I knew she had just made a really bad choice with dire consequences down the road. Ten years later, three more surgeries, and one extra large belly infection, my friend has no abdominal muscles left to support her core and lower back. She can barely walk any distance and her quality of life is very limited at the age of 72. And every day she wants to know, "Why did this happen to me?"

Did any of this have to happen? Do you think she even knows she chose to be in this situation? Is this any different than the person who knows their cholesterol is high, but refuses to do anything about it. Then, voila. Here come the diagnoses: heart disease, bypass surgery, and/or type 2 diabetes? Then it's, "Poor me. Why did this happen?" What about yourself? Take a hard look in the mirror at the health choices you're making right now?

I ask clients all the time to do some basic exercises to help their body heal. I tell them, "If there's anything you can find the time for, it should be core strengthening." Your core (abdominal muscles) supports your gait, your lifting, pulling, sitting, standing, climbing stairs, etc. Most clients say they're too busy, or they're just not interested.

Then one day they go outside, maybe do a little yard work, play some golf, and they get hurt. All because they didn't have the stability to use their body the way they wanted to. As a practitioner, you hope the bells go off, and they start to take better care of themselves, but it's usually not the case.

I tell people all the time, **"YOU CAN'T EXPECT CHANGE IF NO CHANGE HAPPENS." We all make choices that define the direction our life takes.**

We should all take a good look in the mirror and see if we are really viewing life, and ourselves, from a clear perspective. Do you see your spouse for who they are or who you think they are? What about your kids? Are they really the star on the soccer team or just an average player? And, yourself? Now there's a tough one! Are you really an exemplary employee who's doing everything perfectly at work, and the boss just has a personal vendetta against you? Or, are you just seeing it that way? Mirror, mirror, mirror. Every time you take a moment to observe yourself and others, you're now in the moment and not two steps ahead in

136

your thoughts. This is how we begin to see ourselves and the world a lot clearer.

The best example I can give of creating your own reality is with my daughter, Janice, and her ex- fiancé, Justin. Janice and Justin were expecting a baby. Justin really liked to make life what he wanted it to be. As the pregnancy progressed, they would talk about how they wanted to deliver the baby. They were using a mid-wife and wanted a drug-free, natural birth. Since Janice was a nursing student and Justin's mom was a nurse, I asked them what their plans were in the delivery room. "We're going to take the classes, and they told us we would have a nurse with us the entire time to help us through it."

I suggested they might want to do more research and really understand birthing positions, and the labor process, etc. Their response: "We've got it all figured out. The nurse is going to help us with that too." "Oh really," I thought to myself. The next decision was who would be with them when the baby was born. Janice wanted me to do energy work throughout the delivery. Justin was not on board with the energy work, and said I could be there as long as I leave just before the baby was born so they could have that moment together.

I smiled and said to them, "I can be there as a practitioneror I can be there as grandma and to offer support and love and when the baby is being born, I will leave. Or, I told them I don't have to be there at all."

They chose the second option. Janice knew she couldn't have it both ways and as much as she knows the possibilities in my work, selling Justin on it was not going to happen. Together, we decided this was best. Then, the fun began!

Janice went into labor. Now, remember, I'm grandma who's had three C-Sections, never full labor and delivery. My work is quite different; I wasn't well versed in the conventional teachings for breathing and positions during childbirth. I helped the best I could, and lo and behold, there was no nurse to walk us through anything! Justin didn't know how to comfort Janice. He hadn't done any research and intuitive he was not. Janice knew some of the positions, but she couldn't really focus to help us, help her. The contractions were strong and coming fast, but they weren't productive.

This went on for about four hours. I knew the labor was stalled but, remember, my role was Grandma. Why didn't I interfere at that point? My intuition kept saying, "Wait, it's not time yet". But as mom and grandma, I wanted to shake them both like rag dolls! The midwife came to check Janice and she was only at three centimeters. No progression. She decided to medicate Janice so she could sleep through the labor and, hopefully, progress. While Janice slept for a couple hours, Justin's mother, Maureen, showed up.

Janice woke up, the mid-wife checked her, and there was still no progression. They began discussing whether to continue on this path or give Janice Pitocin to progress labor aggressively.

That was my cue! At that moment I said, very loudly, so everyone could hear, "Or." Maureen asked, "Or, what?" I explained what I could do to help everything and as I was explaining, Justin yelled out "We agreed. You're not to get involved." Maureen sent her son out of the room, and asked Janice, "Do you think your mother can help?" "Yes!" Janice replied. Maureen looked puzzled but said to Janice, "It's your body, not his! You get to choose, but Pitocin would be my last choice." I gave grandma-to-be a big smile. Then my daughter finally asked me for help.

I was able to help balance her energy to help her body re-start labor in about 15 minutes. Janice was ready to push in about 45 minutes. She was now pushing and the baby's head was about to crown. At that moment, I realized Justin's wish for everyone to leave the room when the baby was delivered was not going to happen. The baby boy was born with the cord wrapped around his neck, but cried right away, so mom was not worried. While Justin went with the midwife and the baby, I stayed behind to help Janice finish with the cleanup. Everything calmed down, and the midwife brought my grandson to his mother's waiting arms. Mom, dad, and their new baby, it was amazing to watch. As I was packing up and leaving, Justin stopped me as I was almost out the door. He gave me a big hug and a smile and asked me to stay.

Do you think they ever really wanted the first moments alone or did they think that was the way it was supposed to be? I've actually had a couple clients tell me that same scenario. Mom and dad to-be wanted grandma in the room until the baby was

139

ready to be born, but then they wanted that moment alone. Why not do the whole thing alone then? I think I call that conditional support. Do as I say, not as I need. Is there any room for intuition there? Or have we raised a generation of dependent children? Hmmm!

If Janice and Justin had done more homework, they would have had more tools to help each other. Isn't it funny how they planned every moment? Can you really plan life if you're going to live? They knew they would have a nurse and a mid-wife available to them the entire time, and they felt that was such a better option than what Janice has always known and used intuitively.

I was the observer and never interfered until it was needed. All the support they believed was going to be there was not, and the support they didn't want to acknowledge was. For me, it was like a movie playing out to give my daughter a chance to choose her truth with Justin and the accepted norms of society.

What do you think happened to Janice, energetically, at the moment she asked for my help. What happened to Justin when he totally changed his tune and wanted me to stay? Was he sincere? Yes, he was!

I can honestly say everything that happened to Janice and Justin set us up for the next couple of weeks because the baby, Zack, ended up needing emergency surgery. Had they not grown through this childbirth experience, the baby's outcome later on would have been completely different. A little growth goes a long way!

Janice was not the strongest person when she met Justin. After their life experiences together, she is now a very strong, realistic, open minded observer -- and a hell of a nurse. So, was Justin a bad choice or a good choice for her? Ponder that.

Chapter 15
Master Teacher

Rita was in her late 50's. She lived a very healthy lifestyle, but had been struggling with a patch of skin cancer on her right cheek for many years. Her prognosis was not good. She was scheduled for a radical surgery to remove the cancer, leave the wound open, and continue doing surgery until there were clean margins. Rita's doctor told her that she would be very disfigured by the time the desired outcome was achieved.

I saw Rita a month before the scheduled surgery and was able to see that, for some reason, her energy was very imbalanced and her body was not aware of the cancer energetically. Not knowing why, or how, or if this even had anything to do with her illness, I allowed myself to be guided. By the end of the first session, I could tell that her body had reconnected the flow. The body was now aware of the cancer on her cheek. Her energy was working in her favor.

I was happy for her, but also distressed, because I couldn't share this with her for several reasons. What if I was wrong? And if I was right, how could I prove it? I knew in my gut she had been doing self-healing work for a long time and she had made tremendous progress in healing herself. My work just pulled it all together.

After Rita left my office, she had an appointment with her doctor. He was as distressed about the upcoming surgery as she was. He asked her to try an experimental cream for a week to see what would happen. She came back for her third session, and I knew things were really getting better, but I still wasn't comfortable sharing my knowing with her.

You see, I am a complement to medicine. As I do my self-taught energy work, I work with the individual to help them heal themselves physically, emotionally, and spiritually. I guide the individual into finding, and embracing, their own healing. As I explained in Chapter 5 about psychics, I can only read your energy at that moment. If you make different choices when you leave my office, that outcome or energy imprint I read can change directions. My goal is to help you know yourself and how your choices affect your healing. By listening to your Body Within, you will know if your healing is prevailing or not, long before the doctors tell you.

She called me a couple days later to tell me the results of a biopsy performed a week earlier. She explained that a lab had been growing cells to see how aggressive her cancer was. "Everyone is shocked," she told me, obviously elated. "The cancer isn't growing. It's reversing itself. The cream is working!"

I was happy for Rita. The cancer was healing. I knew Rita was healing herself, not the cream. She was in tune with her body and was making choices specific to her and her healing. She wasn't giving away her personal power any more. She was her own healer and had been long before I met her. I was helping her pull it all together.

I talk about how every experience teaches a lesson ... well keep reading! Fast forward five years, and a dear friend and colleague, who had referred Rita, called me. Alice told me that she had just been diagnosed with an aggressive skin cancer on her right cheek and the doctor wanted to do a radical surgery. I was shocked. Wait, it gets better! She asked if I thought I could help her. Alice said her doctor prescribed a cream to try. He said it was a long shot but he had seen it work once before! He hoped Alice would have similar results.

I know what you're thinking... I must have helped Alice and she was cured just like Rita. Wrong. This is the part where life teaches and the art of observation and listening gives you the correct answer - not the answer you want.

As our conversation continued, I refreshed Alice's memory of Rita. I told Alice that Rita was this doctor's other cream patient. Naturally, she was thrilled. This meant I could cure her too! I took a deep breath, and said "Alice, have the surgery." She was floored. She asked me, "Why won't you heal me like you did Rita?" That was Alice's answer. She wanted me to fix her. I explained to Alice that ever since I'd known her she had never healed from inside. Rather, she was always on the bandwagon, gathering quick fixes and empty promises. "If I thought for one second, you had the commitment and self-discipline to heal yourself, I would help you, but there's too much at stake to hope for change." I told her I would be more than happy to help with her post-surgery recovery, which I did. And she had a successful outcome.

Life is the best teacher we all have. I call life, "My master teacher and mentor." Some nights, my daughter, Janice, who is a nurse, comes over. We sit at the dining room table, have a glass of wine, and discuss life. I think of the endless teaching Janice is exposed to on a daily basis, working on a medical surgery floor of a 200-bed hospital. Janice has not only learned from her parents, but also from her time with Justin, her son, her work, etc. I kid around with her some days saying, "Soon enough, you'll be teaching me." We both smile, realizing that, as time passes, we're less mother and daughter and more mentors to each other.

My second child is growing more and more each day. Molly is the most like me. She is energy sensitive and sometimes has trouble adapting to new situations. Molly can feel and sense the energy people give off, not always knowing how to handle it. When I was little, the way I was taught to handle it was to get sent into the fire and let me figure it out on my own. Well, years of lacking self-confidence and fearing others taught me not to do this to her. Again, this is life as the master teacher.

When Molly was younger, I started off by letting her sit on my lap and observe everyone in the room. I explained who everyone was and let her ask questions and come to her own conclusions. From about the age of two to six, it took her anywhere from 15 minutes to three hours before she felt comfortable in a new situation.

145

Then came school age. She did okay, but the first month of every school year was a struggle. Every new teacher and all the new kids around her were a struggle. Not once did I tell her to get over it. I knew what she was going through. Through trial and error, I learned to help her not repeat history. I knew if I could help her understand her thoughts and how they were affecting her experiences, she wouldn't have to struggle so much later in life trying to figure it all out.

Today, Molly is 22, works full time while going to hair styling school, and is the most independent of my three children. We are best friends like I am with my oldest, just in a very different way. Janice helps me deal with life; Molly helps me to be stronger in who I am, to love who I am and who I'm becoming more every day. So, some days I'm the teacher and some days I'm the student. How wonderful is that? This is a perfect example of how life teaches.

I read Dr. Spock when my kids were little. Back then, he was considered "the child rearing bible." It taught me to use intuition and discern what my children needed, and when they needed to graduate from one stage to another.

I remember the bottle was gone as soon as they could hold a cup. The key was if they needed it, it was okay, but if you let them have it past the need stage, they would become emotionally attached. Then it would be much more difficult for them to let go. It was the same with silverware, walking, transitioning to a bed or bedtime, etc.

At each stage of development, if you could just read your children, and what they needed, not wanted, they would just let go when you introduced the next milestone. This taught me so much about watching and listening. They didn't have a bottle past eight months; they walked at 10 months; and were in beds at a year. There were no pacifier issues, etc. I was never mean about it; they ultimately chose it. They just didn't know it.

Now, I watch new mom's struggle. It's not about the child. It's about what the doctor's say, what the books say, or what's convenient for the parents.

If you're a parent, I challenge you to look at your child as an individual. See him or her for who they are and what they need specifically. So many parents parent the way they were parented, or in contrast, boycott the way they were raised. Or they live by something they read. My favorite is, "We don't like society, so we're parenting in a way that boycotts society. Stick it to the man," as they say. Or, are they really just teaching kids to see another fake reality? Let life be your master teacher. Help your kids see what's really happening around them and you'll also become awakened.

Our life experiences teach us how to parent our children, so be sensitive to what is happening in society with kids, schools, and peer pressure. Just because you want to parent a certain way, do your theories fit with what's going on in society? Does it bode well for your child's future?

I had a friend who said her child would never have a cell phone. She felt strongly about their negative influence. I agreed with her, but asked how her daughter would handle not having a phone and being the outcast at school. Well, she said those ever popular words: "She'll be fine. She'll get over it." I smiled and did my thing, then asked if her daughter was strong in who she was, or if she was insecure. Yep, she said it again. She knew where the conversation was going. "She's fine. It has nothing to do with that. She just doesn't need a phone."

So then I asked about mom's high school experience. "Were you strong or insecure?" I asked. Not surprisingly, mom replied, "It's not about that. Society is out of control, and I don't think she should have a cell phone." Maybe, the better approach was for mom to give her daughter a phone but teach her in a way that she figured out for herself that over-use is not good. Use your knowledge to help your kids choose. It may not happen in the first week they have a phone, but you'll see, in time, they'll figure it out if you give them the tools.

Mom's point was valid, but she didn't consider the effects on her child because, in her mind, it didn't matter. Now, if she listened to the news and paid attention to topics like peer pressure, bullying, and teen depression, do you think she might have taken a different approach -- one that didn't isolate her daughter from her peers? Life is happening around her even if mom lives in a chosen reality.

The point I'm trying to make is that life teaches. When we make a decision that will affect us or someone else, we should also look at the effects of the choice from different angles. As soon as you ask yourself, "What is the effect of my choice?" you have to learn a new way of thinking and only then will you realize how big that choice really is.

Every day I'm humbled by things I witness. I have a client and friend who came to me when his dad was dying. Paul loved his dad but didn't do well under this kind of stress. When his dad started to really fail, Paul told me he wasn't going back to see his dad. He wanted to remember him, the way he was.

Well, Paul was completely surprised when I called him a selfish person and told him, "It's not about you." I wish you could have seen his face. I then started questioning him about how his mom and sisters were acting around his dad. He said they were poking and prodding, and basically, driving him nuts. "Well, that really sucks for your dad," I said. "You have a great sense of humor and he adores you and admires your clearheaded thinking. Yet, you're going to let him die with a bunch of women fussing over him pretending he's not dying. What a way to go!"

Paul was very quiet after that, and I wasn't sure how he would handle it, but I said what I said for his dad – and for him. My goal was to break the pattern in Paul's thoughts – to get him to step outside his fear, so he could see another possibility in the situation.

Now, here comes the humbling part. Paul came back and told me that he had been hanging out with his dad, and he broke the ice by making a Top 10 list for his dad to take with him when he meets God. I guess we can thank David Letterman for that one! It was great; I still smile every time I think about it. Paul found a way to make it better, not only for his dad, but for himself as well. Paul's dad went from not being able to talk about dying, to having it all in the open. More importantly, dad's fears about dying diminished and his crossing over was peaceful.

Why is death so hard for us to deal with and talk about? Death is a major part of life. If we take all the experience we've had in life that pertain to death, it gives us tools. Take these tools to re-visit how you feel about death and do you see it with clarity.

As life plays out, we all face death at one time or another. Sometimes it's a loved one, sometimes a friend, even our pets will die. Some are quick and unexpected, some long illnesses. No matter the reason, all of us will die. Life teaches us that we can accept the reality in front of us, or we can pretend something else is happening. Here's a perfect example.

When my mother-in-law Grace was dying, my children were informed every step of the way and weren't shocked when their grandmother eventually died. My kids went to see her in the hospital and as they came out of the room, one by one, they put their arm around me and said "Mom, it's okay. She's ready. She needs to go now. " I had kept them up-to-date on what her doctors said, and when she started to fail. I never kept bad news from them. I told them the truth and let them ask as many questions as they needed to. This not only helped them, but it helped me see things clearer as well.

Another family member, Barbara, took the opposite approach. She protected her children from how bad it was. They were 14 and 16 and had no real understanding of the process. They had no tools and didn't understand the extent of their grandmother's illness. The night Grace died, I took my kids and Barbara's to the hospital café for dinner. The girl asked me when Grammie was coming home. I took a deep breath and said "I'm not sure what you know, but Grammie is not coming home. I'm very sorry, but she'll probably die tonight."

They didn't want to believe me. They just didn't understand what was going on. They asked me several more questions, which I answered truthfully. However, they chose not to believe me. No one else had explained all of this to them, so how could this be? They thought she was fine. My kids tried to help them, but it wasn't their reality; they could only process so much information at once. We went back upstairs to Grace's room and she died within an hour. The girl, who was 16, was so shocked and distraught that she screamed in the hallway. We had to pull her to a private area, and it took her hours to calm down.

Why did this have to happen? Did the parents not know Grace was really that sick? Or, didn't they want to believe it? If they chose not to believe it, how could they tell their kids what was happening? It didn't exist in their world. If, as parents, we don't want to accept what's happening, how can we help our kids?

Sometimes, one person's inability to face life and what's really happening not only impacts them, but it causes a chain of events for those around them. That's why we're all in the dark, to some degree. We started out life as clear souls and then, as our parents teach us about life, do we begin to choose what we believe to be true or just believe what they tell us? As I talked about in Chapter 6, that's how blue prints are established.

Everything that happens to us is an experience. You can choose to learn from it or you can choose to just let life pass you by. I tell people all the time, "If it comes your way – even if it's a homeless person on the street – take a second and reflect. If you feel bad, feel bad. If you feel angry, feel angry. If you feel happy, feel happy and then ask yourself, "Why do I feel this way?"

What this does is help you quantify your thoughts. It helps you realize how you actually view the world. Most people just react with a thought or emotion but don't dig deeper to understand the roots of it. When you really ask, "Why?" you start to truly understand who you are. That, my friends, is how life teaches!

Chapter 16
Answers

Every time you read something, or are exposed to something new, ask yourself "Is it my truth or not?" Do you embrace answers, or do you discard them without consideration because they don't fit with the way you perceive life? I'm equally guilty. When someone gives me advice and it's not what I want to hear, the wall goes up and I never knew the advice was my answer all along.

My husband was out of work. He would search for jobs on the computer, send his resume off into the unemployment abyss and hope for a response. Meanwhile, I would come home with job leads, or someone else would give him a tip, but he wouldn't follow up on it. When I asked why, he would say, "It doesn't work that way. Companies don't want you to send a resume if they're not posting a job." I would and say, "If it comes your way, follow through on it. What do you have to lose? Answers come in many packages, just like motorcycles." ☺ Do you see the connection - or disconnect - in his vision? We're given answers to our questions and problems daily. We just can't see them because they don't look or sound like a Harley!

When I needed shoulder surgery, I got three opinions. Two doctors told me the surgery was risky and not always a good outcome. I wanted the surgery because I was in pain, impatient, and just had it in my head that it would work. I wanted the surgery to be my answer. So I persevered and got a third opinion which was, "It's an easy surgery. I do it all the time, and I have a great success rate." That was definitely what I wanted to hear. So, I did the surgery without giving it a second thought. Well, as I talked about earlier, it didn't turn out so well. The surgeon ended up nicking a nerve and paralyzing muscles in my shoulder which created a lot of right-sided dysfunction.

Could I have seen this coming? Remember, two other doctors felt it was too risky. So, why did I feel the third doctor knew better? Did I use my gut? Hell, no! I didn't even know I had a gut back then. Instead, I discovered that if I push hard enough, I can get anything I want. What I didn't understand back then is what I *want* isn't always what I *need*. It was a very hard lesson for me to learn. Do I regret it? Again, hell no! Why not? Because it made me who I am today!

Answers come in many packages. **Dreams** are one. Dreaming is a great way to ask for help. Sit quietly before you go to bed and ask for an answer to come in a dream. It may take a few nights, and sometimes you remember it. Other times, you remember getting the answer, but don't remember the dream. It will come, just be patient.

Intuition is another. Intuition, a strong knowing, is how most of us get answers. The more you clear away your muck, the stronger the answers become.

154

Synchronicity is another. A series of events just keeps showing up unexpectedly to help you see what you need to see.

People in your life. It could be doctors, teachers, parents, friends, and even total strangers! You never know the package!

Here's another example from my own life that gave me answers. I was having a disagreement with my mom. I try not to let her get to me but this time she did, and I held onto the anger that I wouldn't normally attach to our disagreements. I was out running errands and stopped into the grocery store. An elderly woman was struggling to unzip her coat, so I stopped to help. As I helped with her zipper, she looked confused. Then she realized where she was, thanked me, and went on her way. I didn't give it a second thought until our paths crossed again in the store. She stopped to ask me where they moved the produce department. They didn't move it; she just couldn't find it. At that moment, I knew. With all people in that store, why was I the one to see her distress? I went home and said to my husband, "Someone is trying to tell me to let the argument go. My mom's old and she's not seeing life as clearly as she used to." I did what my gut told me to do and tried to let it go. Three days later I was with my mom and she had an episode that lasted about five minutes. She argued with me about something that happened when she was younger. It was obvious she thought I was someone from her past, and that it was happening now. She was confused and not present. I was stunned. Back in that grocery store, the message came in the perfect package. Even though I acknowledged it, I only saw part of the

155

message until the rest played out. I was sad to see my mom's life heading in this direction, but I was happy to know I wasn't walking alongside her alone.

I also get a lot of my answers in dreams or visions – with a very strong intuition or knowing. As I work with clients to help them clear their energy field, this opens them up to more possibilities, and aids in their overall healing. Some clients start to dream, or have visions. Some develop stronger intuition, and some just become more confident in their knowing. It all depends on their soul's journey. Whatever their soul's strengths are -- that's what gets stronger. There's no specific way for any one person to heal. Some people tell me that other energy practitioners try to put them in touch with their angelic guides. I'm sorry to say that 99% of people live by their gut, not someone talking in their ear. So many people want the process to be cut and dry -- to get an answer from something outside themselves. How is a doctor, parent, teacher, etc., any different than what some perceive to be an angelic guide? Answers are everywhere. The more we become in tune with our surroundings, the more we see, hear and feel our answers.

As I said, dreams play a big part in how I get my answers. Dreams give me yet another tool to work with in dealing with life. I'm going to share a few of my dreams because I want you to know that being aware is not finding bliss and peace for yourself. It's about being aware of what's happening around you and the many tools available to help you handle life. Think of dreams as the same as being a good observer. If you're aware of what's going to happen and you see everyone and everything clearly, without blinders, you always know what's going to happen next. I saw the woman in the store as old and frail. I didn't want to see the true reality of my situation. But once I did, I found peace in an otherwise sad situation. I stopped fighting my reality and sat in it. Peace comes with the release of the fight.

Another example of seeing reality many of us have seen is watching a loved one go down a self-destructive path. When you get the phone call that they're in the ER, and it doesn't look good, you're not surprised. You saw it coming. Of course, you're upset, but not shocked. There's no confusion and you don't fall victim to, "Why or how this could be?" Dreams do the same thing for you. It doesn't make it easier knowing, but it gives you a heads up. And, it helps you understand: We each choose our own path.

Here's an example of my own shifting. I had a dream that was extremely unsettling. At the time, my daughter, Janice, was 4 ½ months pregnant. In my dream I could see her vividly. She was there with the baby and the baby's father. Every time they fed the baby, the food fell out of his mouth. I kept hearing, "The baby can't eat." The only explanation I could come up with was that the baby would be born with a cleft palate, or similar condition. This is where I get into trouble with my intuition. I always have to have a logical explanation rather than waiting to see what happens. The baby couldn't eat wasn't enough for me; I had to give it a diagnosis.

Throughout the pregnancy, I periodically shared my concerns with Janice that the baby was going to have something wrong with it. "He's not going to be able to eat," I told her. "That's all I know." At first, I didn't want to tell her, but my gut kept saying, "She needs to know." At times, she took me seriously and put it in the background and hoped I was wrong – so did I - but at other times she would just say, "Yeah. Okay, mom." I knew from past experience to stay strong and confident in what you know, and it will eventually play out. It may be a day, month or even a year later, but it will play out.

Delivery day came and a perfectly healthy, beautiful baby boy was born. They named him Zack. Janice and I looked at each other. I smiled and said, "I guess I was wrong this time." Happy day! The next day, I spoke to Janice several times. Zack still hadn't taken to nursing. That evening she called to say Zack was undergoing tests to try and determine why he couldn't nurse.

I hung up the phone, rushed to the hospital and sat with the new parents. I had a minute alone with Janice and I asked her "What's your gut telling you?" She said, "Something's wrong – I always felt it, but he's going to be okay." I asked her why she felt it was going to be okay, and she said, "I'm concerned but I'm not scared. I know, mom, I just know. "She asked me the same and I said, "The dream said he couldn't eat, not that he was going to die. My gut feels good. I'm not sure what it could be but let's go with that."

Within three hours, we were being rushed to Dartmouth Hitchcock Medical Center in Lebanon, NH. Tests had revealed that Zack's large and small intestines were not connected. Both the small and large intestines were closed dead ends. We were told it was a very rare condition, but it could be fixed. "He couldn't eat" was the only information I received. How could I know this was the diagnosis? My gut knew I was right, but my brain? My brain wanted more! Let's just say, I'm a work in progress!

Zack had surgery to reattach the intestines, and today he really is a perfectly healthy little boy. Is he perfect because the surgery was a success and the doctors fixed him completely? No. They did the surgery, Zack healed, but then scar tissue became an issue. Janice, who is now a nurse, watched for signs and kept bringing him to me. We tag teamed him, using intuitive energy and body work for the first two years of his life.

Essentially, we read what Zack needed and worked with his body to correct issues as they arose. Fortunately, Zack also has an open minded pediatrician who has helped him heal with some alterative means. The really neat thing about this story is that there wasn't just one answer, but many answers, from multiple modalities that worked together to help Zack. I picked the brains of many alternative and Western practitioners, and used a great deal of intuition. My daughter was also trusting of the process. Her openness, her lack of fear and her ability to make decisions for her son, using all types of medicine still amazes me. I'm 46 and I'm just finding that moxie... I love her for that.

On that note, I challenge those of you in the alternative and Western medicine worlds to consider becoming an ally to one another rather than an adversary. Set aside immediate judgment and really reach out to learn what the other knows. Without many modalities of medicine, this child would not have the life he has today. Ask yourself, "What is it, inside me, which makes me feel my answer is superior?" Why do I feel negative towards the other? Is it because of what you've read, what you think, what you believe? If you sit quietly and ask, I promise, you will get an answer over time. It just may not be in the package you want it in.

Western medicine has divided the body up into so many sections that we don't know how to put it back together! By the same token, Alternative Medicine needs to see the limitations of what they can do, and add to it, the strengths of Western Medicine. There needs to be less criticizing of each other and more respect for what the other brings to the table. When it comes to a practitioner helping a patient, it should be about critical thinking, not personal preferences. If you're a practitioner reading this, and a patient comes in already being treated the opposite of what you treat, feel your internal reaction to what they say. Do you listen with an open mind? Or, is your response to shut the patient down? Did you miss an opportunity to learn from the patient? Think about it. Answers are everywhere!

Another way to get answers is to watch life as it plays out. While my grandson was at Dartmouth, mistakes were made with his care. Not life threatening mistakes, but critical ones none the less. After performing this life-saving surgery, the estimate was it would take seven days to three weeks before they felt his intestines would function and Zack could eat. At three days post op, Zack was looking hungry, had good bowel sounds and clear liquid in the tube from his stomach. The surgeon said if it stayed this way, he could start eating as soon as possible.

An hour later the rounds team of doctors come through, with a totally different diagnosis. They felt it was way too early for Zack's body to be healed, even if it looked like it was. They wanted to put in a central line to feed him for another week. Zack was in distress; he was sucking really hard and crying because he was hungry. It was hard to watch, but it meant he was healing. The parents' heads were spinning. Why another week? What did the surgeon see that these six doctors didn't? Who's right? Mom and dad were just 21 years old. What do they do?

The nurse was not much help because she also thought it seemed way too soon after surgery for Zack to eat. Yet, he seemed ready; all the signs were there. Mom and dad were confused. Who did they trust more at this time? Most of all, what was their gut telling them?

After about two hours of discussion, the rounds team came back to treat Zack, as planned. Justin was tired, weak and unsure of everything up until that moment. He stood up and said, "Don't touch my son. I want to talk to the surgeon." He demanded that the surgeon come. The surgeon came and assessed the situation, looked at mom and dad and said "Let's feed him slow and see how it goes. As soon as he poops and he's stable, he goes home." Well, Zack ate, pooped within the next day and was home that night.

What came over Justin? How did he and Janice get their answers? I just kept asking questions. Questions that made them think – it helped them process what was happening and made them more confident in what they knew. They found their own answers. That's why Justin was so strong at that moment ... his gut took over.

They were two scared kids at the mercy of many credentials. What it took for dad to do what he did was heroic for him. I wasn't sure if either of them was going to step up, but the love for his son and the sight of more needles made Justin trust himself at the deepest level. The answers should have come from the doctor, but they didn't. In this case, they had to find them on their own. I nudged the process but they needed to figure it out and they did. How's that for a package?

More answers came to me as well -- to observe how, even in such a large, respected medical center, care was as divided as alternative and western medicine. You will always have a difference of opinion in medicine so our jobs as patients are to know our bodies and be confident in ourselves and to ask a lot of questions. This is how we find our answers.

Chapter 17
Soul Mates

I was 17, out on my own, and working two jobs. I had just left home and an abusive relationship. I was already learning what it meant to survive. Still, I knew if there was a way to figure out life, I would find it. I had a few friends I could call on for help, but I didn't really know if they would be there for me during the toughest times.

I had met a guy at a few of the pit parties (you would meet at a secluded location and make a bonfire and have fun) that were the rage in my area back in the early 1980s. He and I worked for the same company, so we ran into each other frequently. The last thing on my mind was another relationship, but we stayed friendly. I'm not sure how it happened, but one day I ended up with my ex-boyfriend. We were at a mall that was recently built in our area, and we had a huge disagreement. He left me stranded - no money, no car. I wasn't sure who to call for help.

I couldn't call home, and I didn't have close enough friends I could involve in this mess. I decided to go into the mall and find a pay phone to call this guy from work I hardly knew. Mind you, I didn't have his phone number, and I didn't even know his last name. I had no idea how I was going to find him. I just knew that I had an overwhelming urge to go inside and call him. I walked through the mall entrance, and 15 feet in, there he was, talking

163

with a friend. I stopped in my tracks, not knowing what to say or even think! He saw I had been crying and asked if I was okay. Thirty years later, twenty seven years of marriage... I think I'm okay!

I've always felt that if something inside is urging me to pursue it, even though it doesn't make sense, I should explore it. If I had been overly rational that day, I would never have gone into the mall to call someone whose last name or phone number I didn't know! It just felt right.

Is he my soul mate? I would have to say, "Yes." Are we perfect for each other in every way, see eye to eye on every subject, have all the same likes and dislikes? "Hell, no!" What we do have is a partnership, and a meeting of the minds. Most importantly, we respect each other, even though we don't always agree. We seldom argue because we're able to see each other's side of a situation. We're each allowed to have our own opinion and then come to a mutual agreement. It's about having respect for your partner, and not trying to control one another to make them think like you do.

Have you ever seen a married couple of 20, 30, 40 years? They often look alike; have the same walk; and even some of the same ailments. It's not unusual for them to have the same food likes, the same hobbies, and even the same friends. It's almost as if they're siblings, not a married couple. Why does this happen?

I want you to put both of your hands up in front of you. One hand is the husband's energy, and the other hand is the wife's energy -- or partner, or significant other. Now, slowly move your hands closer together. As they connect and, finally, one covers the other, this is how most married couples live. One person's energy is completely meshed with his or her spouse's energy, so there's very little individual thought left. What I mean by that is not what you may think.

When two people live together, they tend to live in reaction. That is, each partner can anticipate how the other will respond to their actions in a given situation. So, they simply alter their behavior. Over time, the relationship takes on the sound of a well-rehearsed symphony – with each partner careful to play the right tune. In other words, both partners take on pretty defined roles in the relationship. But, here's the problem. When you behave in anticipation of your spouse's reaction, instead of upsetting the situation, or living in it to see what happens, it stops each person from living his or her truth. If one person in the relationship modifies their behavior to appease the other, then the stronger dominates the weaker. The weaker partner's energy is no longer theirs; it's their partner's.

Now, let's look at married couples who don't share any of the same characteristics. First, they don't look alike. They might have some mutual friends but also some of their own. They have separate hobbies and food likes and even very different philosophies on life. They can even agree to disagree! The hands don't cover each other. They stay independent of each other, yet work together. Their energies are separate and blend when they choose to, but they're never influenced by the distortion of their partner's energy.

Which one has a true soul mate?

In my opinion, that would be the second couple. Most people want their partner to think like they think. I wish I had a dime for every conversation I've had with someone trying to make their partner think like they do. Don't get me wrong. There has to be a happy medium with the running of the household, raising kids etc. But the automatic solution to a situation shouldn't be based on how the stronger partner views the world. Rather, the answer should come from both partners asking, "What's the right solution for *this* particular situation?" Who says your glasses see the world more clearly than your partner's?

I look at some of the topics, some of the positions people are trying to get their partners to embrace. Views on life, raising kids, managing money, etc. How many wives follow their husband's lead on these issues? Or, maybe it's the wife who's stronger and the husband lets her choose everything.

Here's another possibility. What if the two of them have a difference of opinion, but instead of the usual weaker-stronger symphony, they decide to strike up a new chord. They discuss the situation openly, and without judgment. Perhaps, they come to the realization that neither is right! "We need to do more research and find a better answer than yours or mine!" The same approach applies to money, food, health and wellness.

Medical decisions. Now, that's a big one. What if one partner decides to use more alternative medicine and take control of their personal health care and wellness? Meanwhile, the other partner uses just western medicine and its theories, and chooses not to help themselves. I find this can really turn a partnership toxic. Beliefs about medicine are equal to religious beliefs. When a partner goes one way, and the spouse doesn't try to see the other's side, life becomes more challenging as a couple.

Wouldn't it be an interesting world if we could live in harmony with someone, and respect their choices, even if we didn't share them? What would we gain? Perhaps, more intellectual stimulation? Someone to challenge our thoughts and beliefs, and open us to new and enlightening ideas? Instead, a lot of couples I've worked with want their partner to think exactly like they do and get upset when they don't!

In most relationships, there's always a submissive person to keep the peace. What do you think happens, on a soul level, if someone sacrifices themselves to keep the peace? In the beginning, it's not too bad. But after 20 or more years of playing this role, we now have two souls meshed into one. That means neither one heals. Plus, the sacrificing spouse is usually the one that gets sick because they have no strength in who they are. Hence, there's no strength to heal. What about when one of the partners die? How does the either one find peace if their energy is nestled together? I talk a lot about clarity and balance. If you live a life with clarity, using intuition - your Body Within, it transfers to dying as well. This is an example of how, if you don't have a strong sense of self in a relationship and are not connected to your Body Within when dying, you might not have the clarity of moving forward peacefully.

Let's look at teenagers. Why do they struggle so much with tangled energies and extreme relationships? Maybe, because it's easier to define themselves by someone else. Take your first love. You have to try it on, see how it fits. If you're strong in your intuition and make choices all the time the love you are experiencing doesn't cloud the brain. If you're not a strong person, you fall prey to using the other person's energy to make you feel whole.

Think about when our kids start to question what we've taught them. Do we tell them *what* to think? Or, do we help them figure out what's best for them in each situation - even when it's not always what's best for us. Maybe if they made more choices as they're growing up, they wouldn't feel the need for someone else in their life to make them feel whole. The more we make decisions for ourselves and learn what we want, the less dependent we are on others to fill those voids within us.

What about your own relationship with your spouse? What cues are your kids picking up? Are you demonstrating that you and your partner are soul mates, or tangled energies? It saddened me many times when my daughter, Janice, was struggling with Justin. He came to me frequently because I talked to him, and I never took sides. Justin wanted to understand how to be an equal partner, not a controlling one. At times, he became very frustrated with me and screamed, "Nobody lives like you people do!" I thought to myself, "How sad is that?" No drama, no arguing. Everyone an equal in the household. Each respecting one another's space in conscious behavior. I really hope this is not as rare as Justin believed.

You see, Justin wanted to be the man of the house, but Janice never thought for a second that there was one person in charge - especially someone in charge of her. Janice found clarity in my space. She heard herself answer my questions and she came to her own realization: She simply wanted more. It was a very challenging part of her journey, as well as mine. As a mom, I could feel her pain. However, if I talked negatively about Justin, it only would have pushed her closer to him. Instead, I just kept asking questions, letting her answer, and she realized she was giving herself the best advice she could receive.

One of the most valuable practices we can develop for our own growth is to listen to ourselves talk. Once we become aware of what's actually coming out of our mouths, we really start to learn who we are, and who we want to become. It's a wonderful gift to give ourselves.

So, why are relationships so important to healing? It all goes back to balance. If you're mindful of balance with exercise, nutrition, rest, etc. but your relationship is still taxing your energy, then you're still out of balance. And, you won't be able to heal.

I've watched a lot of women with cancer not take the proper time for themselves. They continue to take care of everyone and everything in the household. Somehow, they're able to keep up with their treatments and still serve their family. In reality, they're exhausted -- and they're *not* healing. They tell me, "My family can't see that I'm tired, and nobody helps unless I ask, so it's easier to just do things myself." My reply? "If you don't ask, and it's all still getting done, how do they know it's a problem for you? You're still living in the same pattern that got you here."

When is it her time to heal? Why doesn't her family see her struggle? Are they really that blind, or is she really that good at pushing herself beyond her limits?

The risk of living in reactionary relationships, whether it's marriage or with your children, is when you choose to change. When you decide to change your pattern of behavior, your established M.O., make no mistake, it will upset the dynamics in the household. It has to. The person healing will see the need for change, but will anyone else?

I find the biggest obstacle in relationships stems from what I call societal blueprints - patterns of behaviors we pick up from society. Take life sixty years ago, when Mom stayed home and raised the family. Lots of us grew up watching those behaviors. Mom took care of everything and dad went to work. Today, it's more likely that *both* partners work. Problems surface when dad still lives like his dad did, and mom still lives like her mom. It's an unfair balance. I see the struggles of a lot of women. It's a classic reactionary situation. She gets upset, yells, but nobody listens. He doesn't see the problem because his behavior is all reaction to what he saw his dad do. Neither partner has actually observed themselves to see how they react, how they actually behave, and how the house is really run. If they sat with a spread sheet and actually mapped it all out, both would probably be shocked.

Now, take a look at your partner and ask yourself, "Why am I here? Why do I love them? Do I feel like an equal?" If not, ask yourself, "What would make me an equal? Do I treat them like an equal, or do I try to get them to think like me? If they don't share my opinion, do I see why they don't, or do I block it out because it's easier?" Are you walking the path of least resistance?

If you share the same opinion, is it because you both really think the same? Or, is one person simply trying to appease the other? If your husband is trying to appease you, ask yourself, "Why?" If you're the one trying to appease him much of the time, again, ask yourself, "Why?"

Sometimes, a partner's difference of opinion is the best teacher. Think about it. If they see a situation differently, then they just showed you another way to look at life – and maybe offered you some clarity and even more possibilities in your healing.

Hey! Maybe, that's what love is!

Chapter 18
Healing Others While Healing Yourself

I'm sitting in the corner of my treatment room with a client on the table. The lights are very dim and the room is very quiet. I'm discussing the last couple of sessions -- how her reluctance to change, and her unwillingness to abandon the negative path she's chosen, is suffocating her energy.

Why her? Theresa spent many years as a shaman-in-training. Shamanism is a life's work of training the mind, body, and soul. Traditional shamans were tested for strength and endurance for how much they could tolerate in all three areas of who they are. We are Americans; we have no understanding of what that really means. Even from a tribal standpoint, today there are very few true Shamans who understand the depth of knowledge and commitment required to do the healing work they do. We may *think* that we know something is hard, but compare becoming a Shaman to becoming a Navy Seal. There's a reason there are so few of those too!

Theresa went to all the shaman classes and worked with a master, performing countless healings on people. She would be in the room with the master teacher, learning his trade, which dealt with negative energies and emotional issues of all kinds.

Theresa's biggest mistake – her weakness - was that she approached learning shamanism as if she were in a typical classroom. But to be a Shaman, is to commit to a life, not a life style. Theresa saw Shamanism the way she wanted it to be, but never incorporated it into her own healing. This disconnect was overtaking her in an extremely negative way.

The critical piece Theresa missed was that she was supposed to heal with each and every one of her clients. Theresa didn't understand that she was not the healer, but that her role was to be a facilitator of their healing – the facilitator of the joint power and strength she and her client had together.

So, how can you heal yourself while healing others and why do we want to? It's actually easier than you might think. Whenever you're having a conversation with someone, and they seem to be struggling with life, that's your cue to take a step back and really look at who they are, what you know about them, and their choices. Once you're able to see them for who they really are, you can offer advice, or even suggest changes they could make in themselves or their situation to create a different outcome. As soon as you go to that level inside yourself to help others, then you can see the same possibilities in your own life. Theresa overlooked that part, what I call, the mirror of healing.

Many female clients my age come through my office, and most are married to men of the same generation as my husband. Yes, people from the same generation tend to have a lot of the same thoughts and actions, unless they've been awake enough to break patterns and think completely for themselves.

I could put my husband and, at least, four of my friends' husbands in a room, present a scenario, and they would all respond similarly, if not the same. It's an energy imprint of a generation. Take some time to observe your parents and others their age, along with people your own age, and their kids and friends. Sure, there may be some independent thinkers in the mix, but most carry a lot of the same thoughts and theories. Blueprints are not only family generated but society generated also.

How do I heal alongside my clients? As I talk with them about issues they have with their spouses, I mirror my own relationship with my husband. At that moment, I make a choice to reflect on how we live and how we handle similar issues. Do we bury them, or do we discuss them and try to solve them? Every time you observe or talk with someone, it gives you an opportunity to see yourself, for better or worse. It helps you see how far you've come, or how far you still have to go. Mirroring also shows you how many more tools you have than them, or how much more aware of life you are. Just as valuable, sometimes you see how much more aware of life they are than you.

Perhaps, our greatest learning opportunity occurs when you reach out to help someone. You may give them, what you believe, is the answer to their problem. However, they can't see that it's a realistic answer. And, you wonder, "Why can't they see it?" Then you realize there's just no way they can make the changes you're suggesting. This creates a dilemma for you. You may ask yourself, "Why can't they see that all they have to do is make this one change and their life will improve." It's hard for you to process their lack of clarity. When this happens -- and it will, again and again - it should motivate you to look in the mirror. Ask yourself, "Am I seeing reality clearly? Or, is this scenario a healing tool coming to me so that I can see my own reflection. Do I need to make changes and can't or won't?" Ask yourself why.

One day, a client, Rob, told me about a conversation he had with his brother regarding nutrition and exercise. Rob was furious because he felt that all his brother had to do was take his advice and his life would change for the better. Rob kept asking me, "Why won't he listen?" After a few minutes of Rob raising his blood pressure recounting this conversation with his brother, I busted out laughing. Rob looked at me, stunned. I said to him, "What you told your brother was word for word what I've been telling you for two years. Apparently, you really were listening!"

After a few minutes, Rob did better than just see the irony; he saw the clarity. He realized how overwhelmed his wife, and everyone around him, had been by him and his choices, and how ignoring his health was not doing him a service at all. Did he change his habits at that moment? No, but now he knows he has them. Baby steps!

I was talking to yet another person about her struggles with a spouse... how the spouse was very overweight because of poor diet and lack of exercise. She couldn't understand why he wouldn't help himself. Again, I took a step back and asked her, "What did you have for breakfast and when was the last time you exercised?" She replied, "But I'm not overweight." To which I responded, "You're not healthy either. You just have a better metabolism."

The message? Pay close attention to your actions with your kids, spouse, parents, and really take some time to reflect. Is it really about them? Or, are you trying to change them to make them who you want them to be, instead of letting them be who they are? Or, is it possible you're trying to fix yourself by fixing them?

I'll say it again – mirror, mirror, mirror. Whenever you're dispensing advice in an effort to help others, your words will always benefit you if you actually listen to what you're saying!

Chapter 19
Balance Breeds Peace

Lucille was 85 years old. She'd had a wonderful life – a loving husband and seven amazing children. She lived her life and her truth to the max. She had her faith, but she didn't get caught up in the rules or the politics. She used her faith as a guide to help her find her own meaning. Now, the years were catching up with her. Lucille was slowing down, losing her health, and her heart wasn't as strong. Her husband had died two years prior.

Lucille was still living alone, going out with friends, line dancing once a week, and living a productive, whole life. One day, she had a talk with her son and said, "I just want to let you know that I'm good. I've had a great life and I'm tired. I just want to be with your dad." Two weeks later, she went to the doctor. Her heart had kept her going as long as it could, and now it could no longer sustain her. It was quickly breaking down. Lucille was really okay with it; her children were adjusting but also deeply saddened.

In less than ten days, Lucille was in her home, in her own bed, with family surrounding her. She was weak and falling in and out of sleep. Early in the evening, she woke up and asked, "What time is it?" Lucille's daughters replied, "Mom, it's 6 p.m. Lucille looked at them, surprised, and said "Oh my, I've missed my glass of wine before dinner." What were the girls to do? They broke open a bottle of wine, poured everyone a glass, and toasted mom. Lucille took a few sips and fell back asleep. She died just moments later.

Lucille was the mom of a very dear friend. She was also the mom of Paul in Chapter 17 who came to peace with his dad's death by writing the Top 10 list. The changes Paul made through his dad's dying helped mom and his family adopt a clearer vision of death. In turn, this clarity helped their mom to die peacefully. As Paul made choices to listen and observe, he also made choices to change himself and his beliefs. The learning he gained through his mom and dad's deaths raised his energy vibration which will help him and his children throughout life. A single shift of awareness in one person can truly change the outcome for many.

In closing, I urge you to remember all the tools you've accumulated throughout your reading. Use them on yourself daily and really start to open yourself and others to a new and infinite way of thinking. There are lots of people in the world with personal agendas -- to save the Earth, counteract global warming, feed the hungry, etc. My agenda is to get you to look inside yourself. To view yourself and others, and to see where your agenda and your reality lie. Really start to embrace your Body Within. Embrace the messages coming your way. Know that life is an amazing journey filled with choices. Every minute of every day, these choices define the direction our life takes.

As you look around and see the imbalanced energy in the world around you, know that:

CHAOS BREEDS CHAOS.
BALANCE BREEDS PEACE.

Know that bringing balance into your life creates:

Peace in who you are.

Peace in how you live.

Peace when it's time to die.

Here's to you!

May you live a more balanced and peaceful life and may it end with a balanced and peaceful death.

Recommended Reading List

Way of the Peaceful Warrior: A Book That Changes Lives
By Dan Millman

Fools Crow: Wisdom and Power
By Thomas E. Mails

Anatomy of the Spirit
By Caroline Myss

Shaman Healer Sage
Alberto Villoldo

The Joy of Living: Unlocking the Secret and Science of Happiness
By Yongey Mingyur Rinpoche

Signs and Wonders: Finding Peace, Joy, and Direction from
Coincidences, Synchronicities, and Angel Murmurs--and Other
Ways God Speaks
By Albert Clayton Gaulden

Keep Going: The Art of Perseverance
By John M. Marshall III

The Creation of Health
By Caroline Myss

Natural Mandalas: 30 New Meditations to Help You Find Peace
and Awareness in the Beauty of Nature
By Lisa Tenzin-Dolma

Taming the Tiger Within: Meditations on Transforming Difficult
Emotions
By Thich Nhat Hanh

Healing Touch Guidebook, Practicing the Art and Science of
Human Caring

By Dorothea Hover-Kramer

Life After Death: The Burden of Proof?
By Deepak Chopra

Hands of Light: A Guide to Healing Through the Human Energy Field
By Barbara Brennan

The Way of Qigong: The Art and Science of Chinese Energy Healing
By Ken Cohen

Blink: The Power of Thinking Without Thinking
By Malcolm Gladwell

Acknowledgements

I would like to thank my assistant, Heather Riley, for her time and patience in working with me to this project's finish.

Also, my children and my husband for granting me the space to consistently balance myself and my life to make this possible.

I would also like to thank the many clients I have worked with through the years. It has been a hands-on classroom for me, and without their willingness to heal and learn about themselves my journey would have been very different.

I want to give an extra thanks to the key people in my life that have guided me and lent me unconditional support throughout this project and my work.

Thank you!

Virginia Knoetig
Aura Tanguay
Steve Simard
Linda Kaiser
Robert Clegg
Shanna Caron
George Attar
Kathy Garfield
Dana Salb
Heather Riley
Rich Pichette
Tammy Williams
Patricia Quigley

NOTES

NOTES

NOTES

NOTES

NOTES

Made in the USA
Charleston, SC
26 November 2013